Office Procedures in Laryngology

Editor

MILAN R. AMIN

OTOLARYNGOLOGIC CLINICS OF NORTH AMERICA

www.oto.theclinics.com

February 2013 • Volume 46 • Number 1

ELSEVIER

1600 John F. Kennedy Boulevard • Suite 1800 • Philadelphia, Pennsylvania 19103-2899

http://www.theclinics.com

OTOLARYNGOLOGIC CLINICS OF NORTH AMERICA Volume 46, Number 1
February 2013 ISSN 0030-6665, ISBN-13: 978-1-4557-4925-6

Editor: Joanne Husovski
Development Editor: Donald Mumford

Otolaryngologic Clinics of North America (ISSN 0030-6665) is published bimonthly by Elsevier, Inc., 360 Park Avenue South, New York, NY 10010-1710. Months of issue are February, April, June, August, October, and December. Business and Editorial Offices: 1600 John F. Kennedy Blvd., Suite 1800, Philadelphia, PA 19103-2899. Customer Service Office: 6277 Sea Harbor Drive, Orlando, FL 32887-4800. Periodicals postage paid at New York, NY and additional mailing offices. Subscription prices is $335.00 per year (US individuals), $628.00 per year (US institutions), $161.00 per year (US student/resident), $442.00 per year (Canadian individuals), $789.00 per year (Canadian institutions), $496.00 per year (international individuals), $789.00 per year (international institutions), $248.00 per year (international & Canadian student/resident). Foreign air speed delivery is included in all *Clinics*' subscription prices. All prices are subject to change without notice. **POSTMASTER:** Send address changes to *Otolaryngologic Clinics of North America*, Elsevier Health Sciences Division, Subscription Customer Service, 3251 Riverport Lane, Maryland Heights, MO 63043. **Telephone: 1-800-654-2452 (U.S. and Canada); 314-447-8871 (outside U.S. and Canada). Fax: 314-447-8029. E-mail: journalscustomerservice-usa@elsevier.com (for print support); journalsonlinesupport-usa@elsevier.com (for online support).**

Reprints. For copies of 100 or more of articles in this publication, please contact the Commercial Reprints Department, Elsevier Inc., 360 Park Avenue South, New York, NY 10010-1710. Tel.: 212-633-3812; Fax: 212-462-1935; E-mail: reprints@elsevier.com.

Otolaryngologic Clinics of North America is also published in Spanish by McGraw-Hill Interamericana Editores S.A., P.O. Box 5-237, 06500 Mexico D.F., Mexico.

Otolaryngologic Clinics of North America is covered in *MEDLINE/PubMed (Index Medicus), Current Contents/Clinical Medicine, Excerpta Medica, BIOSIS, Science Citation Index,* and *ISI/BIOMED.*

Printed and bound by CPI Group (UK) Ltd, Croydon, CR0 4YY

Transferred to digital print 2012

Contributors

GUEST EDITOR

MILAN R. AMIN, MD
Director, NYU Voice Center; Chief, Division of Laryngology, Department of Otolaryngology, New York University School of Medicine, New York, New York

AUTHORS

PETER C. BELAFSKY, MD, MPH, PhD
Department of Otolaryngology/Head and Neck Surgery, Center for Voice and Swallowing, Davis School of Medicine, University of California, Sacramento, California

CARRIE M. BUSH, MD
Department of Otolaryngology, Georgia Health Sciences University, Augusta, Georgia

MATTHEW S. CLARY, MD
Assistant Professor, Department of Otolaryngology – Head & Neck Surgery, University of California San Francisco, San Francisco, California

MARK S. COUREY, MD
Professor, Division of Voice and Swallowing, Department of Otolaryngology – Head and Neck Surgery, University of California San Francisco, San Francisco, California

MICHAEL M. JOHNS III, MD
Associate Professor, Department of Otolaryngology, Head & Neck Surgery, Emory University, Atlanta, Georgia

MAGGIE A. KUHN, MD
Department of Otolaryngology/Head and Neck Surgery, Center for Voice and Swallowing, Davis School of Medicine, University of California, Sacramento, California

PAVAN S. MALLUR, MD
Department of Otology and Laryngology, Harvard Medical School; Department of Surgery, Beth Israel Deaconess Medical Center, Boston, Massachusetts

ALBERT L. MERATI, MD, FACS
Professor and Chief, Laryngology, Department of Otolaryngology – HNS, University of Washington School of Medicine, Seattle, Washington

GREGORY N. POSTMA, MD
Department of Otolaryngology, Professor, Director, Center for Voice, Airway and Swallowing Disorders, Georgia Health Sciences University, Augusta, Georgia

CLARK A. ROSEN, MD
Professor, Department of Otolaryngology, University of Pittsburgh Voice Center, School of Medicine, University of Pittsburgh, Pittsburgh, Pennsylvania

MANISH D. SHAH, MD, MPhil
Assistant Professor, Department of Otolaryngology-Head & Neck Surgery, University of Toronto, Toronto, Ontario, Canada

C. BLAKE SIMPSON, MD
Professor, Department of Otolaryngology–Head and Neck Surgery, Medical Arts and Research Center, University of Texas Health and Science Center San Antonio, San Antonio, Texas

LUCIAN SULICA, MD
Associate Professor, Director, Laryngology/Voice Disorders, Department of Otolaryngology-Head & Neck Surgery, Weill Cornell Medical College, New York, New York

SEAN X. WANG, MD
Resident, Department of Otolaryngology–Head and Neck Surgery, Medical Arts and Research Center, University of Texas Health and Science Center San Antonio, San Antonio, Texas

Contents

Preface ix

Milan R. Amin

Development of Procedures and Techniques for the Office 1

Matthew S. Clary and Mark S. Courey

This article presents the evolution of current office-based surgery of the larynx, focusing on the development of the tools and techniques for these ambulatory procedures, including laryngoscopy, bronchoscopy, esophagoscopy, and current office-based interventions. Additionally, a historical timeline is presented for the development of office-based laryngology within the context under which laryngology, as a subspecialty, has evolved over the past 200 years, with questions posed to the reader regarding what further developments may arise and how those will affect the practice.

Anesthesia for Office Procedures 13

Sean X. Wang and C. Blake Simpson

The purpose of this article is to provide otolaryngologists with specific instructions on how to adequately perform topical anesthesia for the most commonly performed laryngeal office-based procedures. In this article, patient selection, lidocaine dosing and safety, and patient monitoring are reviewed.

Laryngoscopy, Stroboscopy and Other Tools for the Evaluation of Voice Disorders 21

Lucian Sulica

This article discusses and analyzes the diagnosis and management of voice disorders. Beginning with an insightful description of dysphonia as a sign and symptom rather than diagnosis, and an analysis of its unifying principles, the discussion continues with a review of evaluation, laryngoscopy, stroboscopy, and their respective advantages and disadvantages.

In-office Evaluation of Swallowing: FEES, Pharyngeal Squeeze Maneuver, and FEESST 31

Albert L. Merati

Dysphagia matters and endoscopic examination of patients with swallowing complaints is an important part of their evaluation. The 3 key adjuncts to flexible fiber optic laryngoscopy are (1) flexible endoscopic evaluation of swallowing, (2) assessment of pharyngeal squeeze, and (3) sensory testing. Patients undergoing flexible fiber optic laryngoscopy are then challenged with liquid or solid materials for intake. Fundamental clinical signs of swallowing parameters are noted. The threshold at which the laryngeal adductor reflex is triggered is believed to be helpful in predicting swallowing capacity. This report deals solely with adult dysphagia evaluation.

Transnasal Esophagoscopy 41

Carrie M. Bush and Gregory N. Postma

Since the mid 1900s, esophagoscopy has been performed under sedation or general anesthesia. With transnasal esophagoscopy (TNE), there has been a return to awake, in-office esophagoscopy. Technologic advances have allowed the advent of a ultrathin, flexible esophagoscope that is introduced transnasally, allowing esophagoscopy to be performed in unsedated patients. TNE correlates with conventional esophagoscopy (sedated, flexible esophagoscopy) in diagnostic capacity. Over time, as the benefits of TNE have become elucidated, the procedure has gained wider acceptance and continues to have its role in patient care defined.

Office-Based Botulinum Toxin Injections 53

Manish D. Shah and Michael M. Johns III

Botulinum toxin injections are an effective treatment option for several laryngeal disorders. This article reviews the indications, procedural techniques, potential complications, and outcomes of Botox injections for laryngeal disorders.

Office Airway Surgery 63

Peter C. Belafsky and Maggie A. Kuhn

The emergence and refinement of flexible endoscopes during the second half of the twentieth century has facilitated flexible bronchoscopy's rise as the standard for evaluation of and often intervention in the tracheobronchial tree. Many of these procedures require only topical anesthesia and may be conducted in office settings without sedation. The relocation of procedures previously reserved for the operating room or endoscopy suite confers cost savings, improves provider flexibility, and maintains patient safety while increasing satisfaction and limiting convalescence.

Office-Based Laryngeal Procedures 75

Manish D. Shah and Michael M. Johns III

Awake office-based laryngeal procedures offer numerous advantages to the patient and surgeon. These procedures are well-tolerated, safe, and can be used to treat a wide variety of laryngeal pathology. This article discusses office-based laser procedures and laryngeal biopsies. Indications, procedural techniques, postprocedural care, and potential complications are reviewed in detail.

Office-Based Laryngeal Injections 85

Pavan S. Mallur and Clark A. Rosen

Office-based vocal fold injection (VFI), though initially described more than a century ago, has recently reemerged as an attractive alternative to VFI performed during microsuspension laryngoscopy. Multiple office-based approaches exist, including percutaneous, peroral, and transnasal endoscopic approaches. Surgeon preference typically dictates the approach, although patient tolerance or anatomic variations are also key factors. Regardless of the approach or indication, a myriad of technical considerations make preparation and familiarity requisite for optimal patient outcomes. Office-based VFI offers several distinct advantages over traditional direct or microsuspension laryngoscopy VFI, making it a standard of treatment for a variety of indications.

Index **101**

OTOLARYNGOLOGIC CLINICS OF NORTH AMERICA

FORTHCOMING ISSUES

Endoscopic Ear Surgery
Muaaz Tarabichi, MD,
João Flávio Nogueira, MD,
Daniele Marchioni, MD,
Livio Presutti, MD,
David Pothier, MD, *Guest Editors*

Complementary Medicine in Otolaryngology
John Maddalozzo, MD,
Edmund Pribitkin, MD,
Michael Seidman, MD, *Guest Editors*

Oral Cancer
Jeffrey Myers, MD, Erich Sturgis, MD,
Guest Editors

RECENT ISSUES

Imaging of Head and Neck Spaces for Diagnosis and Treatment
Sangam G. Kanekar, MD
Kyle Mannion, MD, *Guest Editors*
December 2012

Evidence-Based Clinical Practice in Otolaryngology
Timothy L. Smith, MD, MPH, FACS,
Guest Editor
October 2012

HPV and Head and Neck Cancer
Sara I. Pai, MD, PhD, *Guest Editor*
August 2012

Pediatric Otolaryngology: Challenges in Multi-system Disease
Austin S. Rose, MD, *Guest Editor*
June 2012

RELATED INTEREST

Predicting safe tonsillectomy for ambulatory surgery
Original research article by Raja Ahmad, Kahairi Abdullah, Zamzil Amin, Jamalludin A. Rahman
In *Auris Nasus Larynx*. April 2010/Vol. 37, Issue 2

Preface

Advancement of Surgical Techniques Through Technologic Improvements

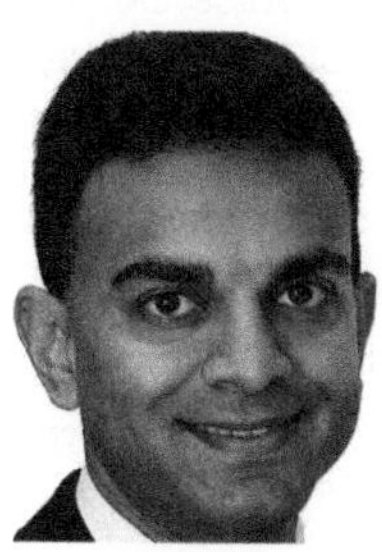

Milan Amin, MD
Guest Editor

There has always been a fascination with technology in Medicine. Throughout the decades, new technology has often been incorporated with the concept that "newer is better." This thought process has often led to great breakthroughs. The implementation process is often very simple. In our own field, the introduction of powered instrumentation to sinus surgery is attributed to a single individual transferring a newer technology used in another field (orthopedics). As is often the case in the history of Medicine, however, many of these ventures into new technology were entered into without forethought into the costs. Witness the multiple forays into the use of "advanced" technologies to remove tonsils. I can remember as a medical student watching a faculty member use a CO_2 laser to perform a tonsillectomy. I can't imagine this was cost-effective.

Nowadays, the business of Medicine dictates that all that we do be scrutinized on the basis of cost. Many hospitals, including our own, factor these issues into the decision-making process when evaluating new technologies for the operating rooms. With the costs of medical care projected to rise far faster than inflation, government agencies and insurance carriers are focusing more intensely on this area.

With that in mind, the topics covered in this edition all focus on advancements in surgical techniques brought about by improvements in technology. The procedures described have, for the most part, been shown to be safe and effective when used for the proper indications. In addition, by moving such procedures out of the operating room, significant cost benefits can be realized over more "traditional" techniques.

One of the goals of this edition is to cover the topic of laryngeal office procedures in a practical and useful manner. The authors have therefore tried to include step-by-step instructions on how they perform them, including tips that are often not included with standard journal articles. We have also included images and video links that will help

Otolaryngol Clin N Am 46 (2013) ix–x
http://dx.doi.org/10.1016/j.otc.2012.11.001

readers learn from the experts who perform these procedures on a daily basis. The hope is that there will eventually be a critical mass of individuals who convert to using these techniques regularly, enhancing the care and cost efficiency of treating patients with laryngeal, pharyngeal, and esophageal problems.

In closing, I would just like to thank the many luminous laryngologists who contributed to this issue.

Milan Amin, MD
NYU Voice Center
Division of Laryngology
Department of Otolaryngology
New York University School of Medicine
345 East 37th Street, Suite 306
New York, NY 10016, USA

E-mail address:
milan.amin@nyumc.org

Development of Procedures and Techniques for the Office

Matthew S. Clary, MD[a], Mark S. Courey, MD[b,*]

KEYWORDS

- Ambulatory surgery • Laryngeal surgery • Surgical procedures • Endoscopy • Laryngology

KEY POINTS

- The dawn of endoscopy began in 1807 with Bozzini.
- Laryngology began in the office in the 19th century, moved to the operating room in the early 20th century, and began moving back toward the office with the advent of improved instrumentation for flexible endoscopy in the late 20th century.
- The collaboration of Harold Hopkins and Karl Storz in 1965, leading to the invention of the Storz-Hopkins telescope, was perhaps the single greatest step toward office-based laryngology.
- Flexible endoscopy has provided the backbone for office-based procedures, including laryngeal injection, in-office laser, and balloon dilation.

INTRODUCTION

Laryngology as a field developed over the course of medical history from the desire to explore the body's internal anatomy and function, that was not readily viewable by external examination. This enthusiasm was guided by both a fundamental desire to understand how people communicated through voice, as well as by the necessity to understand the disease processes that affected the airway and deglutition, thus immediately influencing survival.

Some of the earliest recorded study dates back to the early Greek civilization around 400 BC. The Hippocratic School had a basic understanding that the epiglottis helped protect liquids from entering the pharynx. During the Roman era, dental mirrors

Financial disclosures: None.
Conflicts of interest: None.

[a] Department of Otolaryngology - Head and Neck Surgery, University of Colorado, 12631 E. 17th Avenue. B-205, Aurora, CO 80045, USA; [b] Division of Voice and Swallowing, Department of Otolaryngology – Head and Neck Surgery, University of California San Francisco, 2330 Post Street, 5th Floor, San Francisco, CA 94115, USA
* Corresponding author.
E-mail address: mcourey@ohns.ucsf.edu

Otolaryngol Clin N Am 46 (2013) 1–11
http://dx.doi.org/10.1016/j.otc.2012.08.013
0030-6665/13/$ – see front matter

were being used to explore the oral cavity. Galen provided the names for the epiglottis and the recurrent laryngeal nerve in the second century AD.[1]

This interest in endoscopic exploration continued through the Renaissance period with Julio Casserius, whose book titled "The Anatomy of Voice and Hearing" in 1600 AD detailed the laryngeal anatomy of mammals including people.[2] During the turn of the 19th century, Anderesch, Swan, and Henle were involved in detailing the early neuroanatomy of the larynx, as well as its histology.[3] Dutrochet, in 1806, communicated some early theories on passive vibration of the vocal folds to generate sound despite never having observed a functional larynx.[2]

These early times set the stage for the explosion of technology and understanding of laryngeal function that occurred during the 19th and 20th centuries and continues today. Continuous efforts to improve visualization of laryngeal anatomy were the driving force for the creation and evolution of the field. Endoscopy and the stepwise improvements in endoscopic technology have provided the trunk from which operative interventions have been able to sprout.

Laryngologic surgery, as a result, evolved from office-based procedures to operating room surgery, and then back toward office-based surgery in the current day. This process occurred in a gradual but discretized fashion through the contributions of many people over the course of 200 years. It is easy to be unaware of or to forget the arduous course that the field has taken to get to the point where surgery on the aerodigestive tract can be performed in the awake patient in the office setting. It is important to understand the history of technical developments and practice so that one can continue to move forward. This article attempts to describe that course.

ENDOSCOPY EARLY YEARS

The field of endoscopy began to take root in 1807 with Philip Bozzini. In an effort to view the internal anatomy, Bozzini developed several speculae to explore the different human orifices. He was the first to use an external light source, in the form of candlelight channeled by mirrors, to visualize the internal body. He is not believed to have observed the larynx, but he did advance the entire field of endoscopy.[4] The early attempts at visualization of the larynx were all variations of indirect laryngoscopy using a system of rudimentary mirrors to reflect the image back to the observer while attempting to channel light down to the larynx. Benjamin Babington is credited with developing the first "Laryngoscope" in 1829. With the patient in sitting position, Babington's device retracted the tongue to allow the larynx to be visualized by a mirror, while illumination was provided by external direct sunshine. His efforts were subsequently forgotten due to a lack of publishing clinical papers.[5] In 1841, Friedrich Hoffman developed the perforated concave mirror that is classically associated with the otolaryngologist.[6] Avery used a concave mirror affixed to his head to reflect candlelight in conjunction with Bozzini's scope in 1846. In 1855, Avery was the first to place a curved mirror on a headband, thus freeing both hands to examine the patient.[5]

Manuel Garcia, a music professor, is oftentimes credited with being the first to perform indirect laryngoscopy. Garcia used a device similar to Babington's to examine his own larynx but did not publish his work until 1854, several years after other investigators. In 1855, he published "Observations on the Human Voice," in which he described vocal fold motion, as well as the generation of voice from the vocal folds. He was the first to describe the concept of the autoscopic laryngeal examination.[2,7]

After the advent of tools that allowed for endoscopic views of the larynx, efforts began to apply these developments to the clinical setting. The first laryngology clinic was established in Vienna in 1870 by Von Schroetter. During this period, indirect laryngoscopy faced several technical hurdles. Both lighting for visualization and laryngeal anesthesia had always been formidable challenges to examination. Thomas Edison's invention of the electric incandescent light bulb did not occur until 1879, and topical anesthesia for the larynx was not discovered until 1884. As a result, it was difficult to establish indirect laryngoscopy for everyday use in the laryngology clinic. In 1884, Koller discovered the use of cocaine for ophthalmic topical anesthesia, and Jelinek was the first to apply it to the larynx to remove a polyp.[2] Before topical anesthesia, laryngeal examination required the process of habituation by the patient to overcome the gag reflex and laryngeal stimulation. Johann Czermak was the first to employ artificial light with a curved mirror to concentrate the light source, as he described in 1888.[2,8] Czermak continued to perfect techniques and tools for indirect laryngoscopy to establish clinical relevance. He helped to educate many physicians at the time in indirect laryngoscopic operative techniques, notably Jacob Solis-Cohen.

Morell MacKenzie, also a student of Czermak, helped to establish the first hospital for throat diseases in the late 1800s. He was also the first to coin the term laryngoscope, although the devices that he used were still forms of indirect "Laryngoscopy" that reflected the image back to the examiner. MacKenzie spent considerable time improving and developing instruments for laryngeal examination and biopsy. He also authored the first textbook of throat diseases.[7]

Most laryngology endeavors took place in Europe, until Horace Green brought the field to North America. He is touted as the father of American laryngology. Having completed his studies in Paris, Green immigrated to the United States and brought the field with him. Green had several significant accomplishments, including being the first to excise a laryngeal neoplasm under direct laryngoscopy using a spatula and curved tenaculum.[9,10] He also was the first to introduce medication into the larynx and bronchi for treatment of local disease.[11] In the middle of the 19th century, the practice of laryngology was performed by medical physicians and neurologists. Jacob Solis-Cohen, a general surgeon, helped to initiate the transition of the field into a surgical specialty. He was among the first surgeons to focus on the larynx and is believed to have performed the first viable total laryngectomy in 1884.[12] During the same period, airway obstruction, often due to foreign bodies, was being treated surgically with tracheotomy or by cannulation of the larynx using indirect laryngoscopy.[13]

THE ADVENT OF DIRECT ENDOSCOPY

These efforts in the 19th century opened the door for the contemporary field of endoscopy, which was coined by Antonin Desormeaux, a urologist, in 1853.[14] Once clinical utility was established, the field and the technology were able to progress much more rapidly. Development of direct laryngoscopy, bronchoscopy, and esophagoscopy occurred very much in parallel with each other through sharing of technical leaps. Kussmaul performed the first the direct esophagoscopy in 1868. His concept for esophagoscopy was taken from studying sword swallowers and then applied using the Desormeaux urethroscope to evaluate the esophagus.[15] In 1881, von Mikulicz developed the first electrically lighted esophagoscope using a platinum burner. However, it wasn't until 1888 that Leiter replaced the burner with the incandescent light bulb for use with endoscopes.[16] Having developed a strong enthusiasm for von Mikulicz's esophagoscope, Alfred Kirstein is given credit for the developing the first true direct laryngoscope. The introduction of his device in 1895 ushered in a new era of modern diagnostic and operative laryngology. Interestingly, his "Autoscope", as he called it, was described in the first issue of the *Laryngoscope* journal.[1,2] In 1896, Gustav Killian was active in researching the possibility of using rigid scopes to explore the trachea and bronchi.[17] Previously, Green had demonstrated that the subglottic airways down to the lungs could be instrumented. It was believed that if esophagoscopy could be tolerated safely, then bronchoscopy should be feasible. Killian was the first to demonstrate that airways could be safely explored by passing a 9 mm tube beyond the carina. He introduced the supine position and coined the term "Bronchoscopy".[18]

Chevalier Jackson designed his first laryngoscope in 1903. At the time, endoscope designs incorporated variations of spatulas and tubes to aid displacement of oral and pharyngeal structures. Jackson developed tubed designs for his laryngoscopes, bronchoscopes, and esophagoscopes. This design allowed for advancement of the scope through a more lateral approach, providing better distal exposure without obstructing the view. However, closed-tubed endoscopes conducted the standard proximal light source poorly. To find ways to deal with poor lighting, innovators began experimenting with distal lighting for endoscopes. Although it had been introduced previously in Europe, Chevalier Jackson is credited with developing a practical distal lighting method for endoscopy equipment in 1905. He used a side channel (tube within a tube concept) on his scopes to accommodate the light. In addition, he also introduced distal suction. He devoted a great deal of thought to patient positioning, as well as arrangement of equipment and personnel during procedures.[12,17,19,20] In order to facilitate his operative setups, endoscopy was moved to the operating room. This transition to the operating room likely set the stage for future technology adoption.[21]

With the advent of direct laryngoscopy, it became clear that laryngeal surgery could benefit from bimanual techniques. Killian introduced suspension laryngoscopy in 1911 serendipitously for the purpose of stabilizing the scope on the patient's chest to draw better diagrams of the larynx.[2,22] Lynch then made modifications to Killian's apparatus, which helped to bring about its adoption in the United States. In 1920, he published the first series of early glottic cancers resected using direct laryngoscopy.[23] Yankauer began to use magnification for endolaryngeal surgery but recognized the limitations of monocular vision. In 1910, Yankauer introduced a laryngoscope that was wide enough to permit binocular vision, but it did become popular until the widespread use of the binocular microscope.[24] Edwin Broyles introduced bronchoscopes with magnification in the 1940s.[25] Multiple scientists devoted time and effort to both improving magnifying telescopes as well as surgical techniques. These helped to develop the art of bimanual manipulation of the larynx.

THE OPTICAL ERA

The state of endoscopy in the 19th and early 20th centuries was dictated by the lack of magnification of distant structures and inadequate visualization from poor lighting. Over the course of the past century, a quantum leap in endoscopic technology allowed for further development of the field of laryngology as well as the movement of surgical intervention from the operating room back into the office.

The 1950s were marked by significant advances made in optics and illumination. The advances in these areas occurred in tandem and were enablers for today's surgical practices. In 1953, the Zeiss Optical Company introduced the binocular microscope.[26] The coupling of a microscope with endoscopes was initially proposed for gynecologic applications. During the second half of the 1950s, Albrecht and Kleinsasser in Europe and Jako in the United States began exploring possible uses of binocular microscopy in the larynx.[27] In 1960, Scalco described the use of the Zeiss microscope with the Lynch suspension laryngoscope.[28] Binocular microscopes necessitated redesign of laryngoscopes to take advantage of stereoscopic vision.

Also in 1960, Kleinsasser developed instruments for use under binocular microlaryngoscopic conditions. He introduced a laryngoscope that used warm air to keep the telescope from fogging, since cuffed endotracheal tubes were still not being used for laryngoscopy at that time.[29] The 1970s saw the introduction of fiberoptic light carriers to replace distal incandescent light bulbs, along with laryngoscope redesign by Jako and Dedo. The advances in technology allowed Von Leden to create the modern technique of laryngeal microsurgery in the 1960s.[26]

Further improvements in endoscopic image transfer were occurring simultaneously with advances in direct microlaryngoscopic techniques. In 1959, the rod lens optical system was invented by Harold Hopkins. His design used a glass rod to replace the air interspace between lenses of the existing telescopes at the time. The new optical design provided a wider viewing angle and absorbed less light during image transmission down its length.[30,31] Interestingly, his invention received very little interest. Meanwhile Karl Storz, having observed the prototype for the flexible fiberglass gastroscope in 1960, realized the potential for using fibers to carry light. He began developing the idea of coupling a fiberoptic light source with rigid telescopes. His technology was a marked improvement over Jackson's distal illuminating bulbs, which were not only dim but highly unreliable and would frequently burn out during the case.[31] Before this, Storz had been involved in the development of instrumentation for otolaryngologic applications. He was familiar with the limitations of the current lighting and optic systems and recognized the need for improvement in both to provide better endoscopic visualization. Storz arranged to meet with Hopkins in 1965. The two partnered and quickly developed the Storz-Hopkins telescope.[31] Their scope provided superb image resolution with unmatched illumination. This provided a marked improvement in the quality and ease by which to acquire clinical photography. Aside from its role in the operative theater, it also improved the ability to share and collaborate with others in the field on clinical problems.

THE BEGINNING OF CONTEMPORARY OFFICE-BASED ENDOSCOPY

It is important to recognize that until the 1960s, endoscopy was generally performed only with rigid instruments and in awake patients. General anesthesia with mechanical ventilation as it is known today was critical for the evolution of airway sharing between anesthesia and otolaryngologist. Due to general anesthesia, endoscopy with rigid techniques was better tolerated and thus aided its movement from the office into the operating room. However, as techniques of flexible indirect endoscopy developed from advances in fiberoptic lighting and image transfer, it became possible to again perform certain procedures with little or no anesthesia. As with rigid endoscopy, initial flexible endoscopy was used in other medical disciplines before being adopted by otolaryngology. Edward Benedict introduced flexible gastroscopy to the United States in 1933 using the Wolf-Schindler gastroscope, which was developed in 1932.[32] The early flexible scopes were rigid proximally and flexible distally to allow for accommodation around the internal anatomy of the patient. The optic systems were composed of a complicated series of lenses inside the scope that provided very poor image quality. Flexible endoscopy developed from the work of John Tyndall, who in 1870 first described the optical properties of glass rods, which allowed light to be guided. Further development in optical light and image technology by Baird and Hansell incorporated light-guiding properties from glass rods into glass or plastic fibers. These optical fibers were stretched until they were long, thin, and flexible. Heinrich Lamm suggested that bundles of optical fibers could be used in flexible scopes in the 1920s.[33,34] Optical bundles were further improved with the inclusion of glass-clad fibers. In glass-clad fibers, each fiber has a protective coating with a lower refractive index that decreases interference between fibers, and subsequently decreases attenuation of the image as it travels down the fiber.

These technologies led to the creation of the first completely flexible endoscopes. In 1957, the flexible fiberoptic gastroscope was introduced by Hirschowitz and Curtiss, and was 0.5 in in diameter.[35] From that time on, fiberoptic instruments have been developed for gastrointestinal (GI) applications first, and then with miniaturization of the devices, new uses for the technology develop. In 1963, Howard Andersen performed the first transbronchoscopic lung biopsy using a Holinger flexible forceps through a rigid bronchoscope. The first flexible bronchoscope was introduced by Ikeda in 1966. Flexible instrumentation developed in conjunction with the enlargement of the side channel.[34] Swashima and Hirose were the first to describe the flexible fiberscope in 1968, which was the first flexible transnasal endoscope.[36] This allowed laryngology to move from mirror-based indirect laryngoscopy to fiberoptic laryngopharyngoscopy. This sentinel event truly opened the door for office-based laryngology as it is known today.

After the advent of the flexible fiberoptic laryngoscope, chip tip technology was the next advance to impact the field of laryngology. The charge-coupled device (CCD) was invented in 1969 at AT&T Bell Labs (Berkeley Heights, NJ).[37] This technology was incorporated into image capture devices for the first time in 1975 and provided a marked improvement in the quality of photographs through digitization of the presented image. Three CCD cameras, which followed the 1-chip devices, use a dichroic beam splitter prism to divide image colors and provide better resolution and contrast.[38]

As with fiberoptic scopes, CCD technology found its way into GI applications first. The first scope was introduced by Welch Allyn in 1984 for GI applications.[39] In 1987, the first chip made its way into a flexible bronchoscope by Ikeda and then became commercially available in 1990.[18] By the 1990s, CCD technology had improved enough to allow the production of chips with resolution approaching that of the rod–lens telescope. In addition, the size of the chips became small enough to allow passage comfortably through the nasal cavity. Finally in 1999, the chip tip transnasal endoscope was introduced for applications in otolaryngology. These endoscopes combined a CCD camera for image transfer with fiberoptic technology for light transfer. It was first used for transnasal esophagoscopy (TNE), and then for nasopharyngolaryngoscopy (NPL).[40] Leisser was the first to describe going through the nose with a gastroscope in 1990. This was performed in a patient with an altered mental status and unwillingness to open his mouth.[41] In 1993, Shaker described the feasibility of TNE with a fiberscope for clinical evaluation.[35] Dean and colleagues[42] showed in 1996 that TNE was comparable to traditional esophagogastroduodenscopy. Koufman was the first to describe the technology in the otolaryngologic literature in 2001 using the 5.1 mm chip tip scope.[43] This is where endoscopy stands today.

FLEXIBLE ENDOSCOPY: A MEANS TO AN END

Advances in endoscopic technology provided a means by which to potentially transfer laryngologic procedures from the operating room back into the office setting. The first laryngeal-based intervention to be moved into the office was injection laryngoplasty. Before Arnold's description in 1955, there was no treatment for vocal fold paralysis. Isshiki introduced medialization thyroplasty in 1974.[44] Brunings attempted vocal fold injection with paraffin in 1911, but the injectable extruded as well as caused paraffinomas, and the technique was essentially forgotten.[45] Arnold reintroduced the injection laryngoplasty in 1955 through a laryngoscope using autogenous tissue.[46]

In 1962, he suggested Teflon paste due to injectability, tissue tolerance, and lack of resorption. Dedo described his series of 135 patients in 1973, who were injected with Teflon transorally while awake using mirror indirect laryngoscopy with a Brunings' syringe.[47] Ford was the first to propose collagen injection in 1984, due to ease of injectibility and temporary nature.[48] It was not until 1985, when Paul Ward introduced the technique of transcervical injection, that the current office-based technique came into being.[49] Currently, there are numerous variations of the transoral and transcervical techniques as well as injectable fillers that can be used in the office setting.

Laser Technology in Office-based Laryngeal Surgery

Office-based laser surgery has also been advanced by the development of laser technology. As miniaturization of flexible endoscopes continued with smaller chips and improved lighting, the addition of working channels was able to be accomplished. At the same time, advances in laser delivery systems including the introduction of wave guides for carbon dioxide (CO_2) laser facilitated the safe use of lasers even in awake patients. The laser was invented in 1958. Pulsed laser systems had been used for otologic applications before their use on the larynx. In 1965, Jako began looking at its use on the vocal folds. He trialed lasers of multiple wavelengths but found that the CO_2 laser had the optimal depth of penetration. The first endoscopic laser delivery system was developed in 1968 for use with the binocular microscope.[50,51] A coupling device for the rigid bronchoscope was created. Stuart Strong then began using the CO_2 laser for the extirpation of papilloma through a bronchoscope in 1972.[18] In the same year, Strong and Jako began resection of early laryngeal cancers with the CO_2 laser. This was performed through binocular endoscopic visualization, combined with the use of a micromanipulator on the operating microscope.[52] In 1974, Strong published a series of 11 patients with midmembranous vocal fold lesions treated with the CO_2 laser.[53] The early reports were still performed using rigid techniques, and by the early 1970s, they were commonly performed under general anesthesia. The role of lasers in surgery continued to increase when Dumon introduced the use of Nd-YAG laser in bronchoscopy in 1980.[54] The CO_2 laser was the standard of care for treatment respiratory papilloma until 1998, when McMillan proposed using the 585 nm pulsed dye laser (PDL). He based his work off of Anderson and Parrish's concept of selective photothermolysis from 1993 and Tan's work suggesting that the PDL may be useful for the treatment of cutaneous warts by coagulating blood vessels at the microvascular level.[55,56] He suggested that the PDL was the ideal laser for patients requiring repeat surgeries, because he believed it provided better control of ablative depth.[57] At the same time, a better understanding of pulse structure and the development of computerized micromanipulators for the CO_2 lasers occurred. This allowed precise ablation of epithelial disease with minimal unwanted surrounding thermal injury. The advantage for PDL was that it could be delivered through a flexible fiber that would fit through the channel of a transnasal endoscope. This allowed the procedure to be done without sedation or general anesthesia. The indications for PDL expanded in 2003 when it was first used for glottic dysplasia in the operating room setting by Franco and colleagues.[58] Once this approach to laryngeal lesions was demonstrated to be practical, it was transferred to the office setting. Zeitels described the first series of office use of PDL in 2004 using a flexible scope to treat both laryngeal dysplasia and papillomatosis.[21] Also in the same year, the hollow-core CO_2 laser fiber was introduced, thus transferring a heavily used surgical modality from the operating room to the office. In its first application, it was used by Koufman to treat papilloma at the carina.[40] The 532 nm potassium titanyl phosphate (KTP) laser was introduced in 2006 for use in the office because of its improved hemostatic properties as compared with the PDL.[59] These advances in both instrumentation and techniques opened the door for the ever-expanding applications for office-based surgery with the laser.

Dilatational Methods in Airway Surgery

Practical and safe awake airway and esophageal dilation came into wide use only recently during the 2000s due to the introduction of flexible endoscope. As early as 1871 in Europe, Von Schroetter developed 2 dilational methods specifically for the airway. One system used hard rubber bougies that were introduced through the mouth, while the other involved curved metal dilators that were passed through a tracheotomy.[60,61] These systems were used well in advance of general anesthesia and even topical anesthesia. O'Dwyer used a similar technique in the United States in 1888 that required daily dilation of the airway.[62] Henry Plummer was the first to introduce the concept of a guide wire by using a silk thread as an aid to esophagoscopy in 1910.[63] Dilational techniques for the airway and esophagus continued to evolve. Jackson developed triangular shaped dilators in the early 1900s for dilation of the glottic aperture. In 1915, Hertz introduced his rubber dilators for the esophagus. Maloney modified them in 1960 to include a tapered end, which brought them into the form that most are familiar with today.[64,65] Bougie dilation was the standard for esophageal applications until 1981, when Gruntzig balloon catheters were first described in the gastroenterology literature for dilating strictures.[66] Balloon dilation was accepted as a viable alternative to bougienage, while controlled radial expansion balloons began to be produced specifically for these types of applications. In 2007, balloon dilation of the esophagus made its leap to the office. Rees[67] introduced unsedated transnasal balloon dilation of the proximal esophagus. The series in 2009 demonstrated the feasibility and safety of esophageal procedures being performed in the office.[68]

SUMMARY

The field of laryngology and office-based procedures has traversed a long course from the early 19th century to the practices of the current day. It is easy to take for granted the tools and techniques that are used daily without reflecting upon their impact on the ability to care for patients. When one reflects on their development, one is better able to appreciate the curiosity and ingenuity that led to the contemporary practice of laryngology. This reflection may help in the stepwise march forward. The future will allow one to dictate which questions need to be asked and how they will be answered. How will the delivery of medications to the larynx evolve? Will traditionally invasive procedures continue to move from the operating room to the office? What instruments will be needed to allow 2- handed instrumentation in the outpatient setting? How can in-office endoscopy be improved, and what discoveries will ensue? Through reflection of the history of office-based laryngology, one can hopefully continue its progression into the future.

REFERENCES

1. Assimakopoulos D, Patrikakos G, Lascaratos J. Highlights in the evolution of diagnosis and treatment of laryngeal cancer. Laryngoscope 2003;113(3):557–62.
2. Alberti PW. The history of laryngology: a centennial celebration. Otolaryngol Head Neck Surg 1996;114(3):345–54.
3. Alberti PW. The evolution of laryngology and laryngectomy in the mid 19th century. Laryngoscope 1975;85:288–98.
4. Reuter HJ. Philip Bozzini and endoscopy in the 19th century. Stuttgart (Germany): Max Nitze Museum; 1988.

5. Mackenzie M. The use of the laryngoscope in diseases of the throat. Philadelphia: Lindsay and Blakiston; 1865. p. 9.
6. Hofmann O, Brusis T. On the origins of the first German otorhinolaryngology (ORL) clinics. J Laryngol Otol Suppl 2005;30:41–4.
7. Rosenberg PJ. Total laryngectomy and cancer of the larynx. Arch Otolaryngol 1971;94:313–6.
8. Bryce DP. The American Laryngological Association, 1878–1978: a centennial history. Washington, DC: American Laryngological Association; 1978.
9. Green H. Morbid growths within the larynx. In: On the surgical treatment of polypi of the larynx, and oedema of the glottis. New York: G.P. Putnam; 1852. p. 56–65.
10. Elsberg L. President's address: laryngology in America. Trans Am Laryngol Assoc 1879;1:30–90.
11. Snyder C. The investigation of Horace Green. Laryngoscope 1975;85:2012–22.
12. Weir N. Otolaryngology: an illustrated history. Boston: Butterworth-Heinemann, Ltd; 1990.
13. O'Dwyer J. Chronic stenosis of the larynx treated by a new method, with report of a case. N Y Med Rec 1886;29:641.
14. Desormeaux AJ. The endoscope and its application to the diagnosis and treatment of urinary affections. Chicago Med J 1867;24:177–94.
15. Becker HD. Gustav Killian, a biographical sketch. J Bronchology 1995;2:77–83.
16. Berci G. Endoscopy. Englewood (CA): Appleton-Century- Crofts; 1976.
17. Jackson C. Tracheo-bronchoscopy, esophagoscopy, and gastroscopy. St. Louis (MO): The Laryngoscope Co; 1907.
18. Marsh BR. Historic development of bronchoesophagology. Otolaryngol Head Neck Surg 1996;114:689–716.
19. Hawkins JE, Schacht J. Sketches of otohistory: part 7-the nineteenth-century rise of laryngology. Audiol Neurootol 2005;10:130–3.
20. Weir N. History of medicine: otorhinolaryngology. Postgrad Med J 2000;76:65–9.
21. Zeitels SM, Franco RA Jr, Dailey SH. Office-based treatment of glottal dysplasia and papillomatosis with the 585-nm pulsed dye laser and local anesthesia. Ann Otol Rhinol Laryngol 2004;113(4):265–76.
22. Jackson C. Peroral endoscopy and laryngeal surgery. St. Louis (MO): Laryngoscope Co; 1915.
23. Lynch RC. Intrinsic carcinoma of the larynx, with a second report of the cases operated on by suspension and dissection. Trans Am Laryngol Assoc 1920;40: 119–26.
24. Lewy RB. Depth perception in laryngoscopy. Arch Otolaryngol 1960;72:383–4.
25. Carroll GG. The laryngeal microscope and bronchoscopic and esophagoscopic telescope. Trans Annu Meet Am Bronchoesophagol Assoc 1932;19–21.
26. Nogueira JF Jr, Hermann DR, Américo Rdos R. A brief history of otorhinolaryngolgy: otology, laryngology and rhinology. Braz J Otorhinolaryngol 2007;73(5):693–703.
27. Von Leden H. The history of phonosurgery. In: Sataloff RT, Gould WJ, editors. Voice surgery. St. Louis (MO): Mosby-Year Book; 1993. p. 74–9.
28. Scalco AN, Shipman WF, Tabb HG. Microscopic suspension laryngoscopy. Ann Otol Rhinol Laryngol 1960;69:1134–8.
29. Jako GJ. Laryngoscope for microscopic observation, surgery, and photography. The development of an instrument. Arch Otolaryngol 1970;91(2):196–9.
30. Berci G, Kont LA. A new optical system in endoscopy with special reference to cystoscopy. Br J Urol 1969;41(5):564–71.
31. Linder TE, Simmen D, Stool SE. Revolutionary inventions in the 20th century. The history of endoscopy. Arch Otolaryngol Head Neck Surg 1997;123(11):1161–3.

32. Benedict EB. Examination of the stomach by means of a flexible gastroscope: a preliminary report. N Engl J Med 1934;210:669–74.
33. Van Heel AC. A new method of transporting optical images without aberrations. Nature (Lond) 1954;173:39.
34. Ikeda S. Atlas of flexible bronchoscopy. Tokyo: Igaku Shoin; 1974.
35. Shaker R. Unsedated trans-nasal pharyngoesophagogastroduodenoscopy (T-EGD): technique. Gastrointest Endosc 1994;40(3):346–8.
36. Sawashima M, Hirose H. New laryngoscopic technique by use of fiber optics. J Acoust Soc Am 1968;43(1):168–9.
37. Janesick JR. Scientific charge-coupled devices. Bellingham: SPIE Press; 2001.
38. Dobbin B. Kodak engineer had revolutionary idea: the first digital camera. Available at: seattlepi.com. Accessed on November 15, 2011.
39. Classen M, Phillip J. Electronic endoscopy of the gastrointestinal tract. Initial experience with a new type of endoscope that has no fiberoptic bundle for imaging. Endoscopy 1984;16(1):16–9.
40. Koufman JA. Introduction to office-based surgery in laryngology. Curr Opin Otolaryngol Head Neck Surg 2007;15(6):383–6.
41. Leisser A, Delpre G, Kadish U. Through the nose with the gastroscope. Gastrointest Endosc 1990;36(1):77.
42. Dean R, Dua K, Massey B. A comparative study of unsedated transnasal esophagogastroduodenoscopy and conventional EGD. Gastrointest Endosc 1996; 44(4):422–4.
43. Belafsky PC, Postma GN, Koufman JA. Normal transnasal esophagoscopy. Ear Nose Throat J 2001;80(7):438.
44. Isshiki N, Morita H, Okamura H, et al. Thyroplasty as a new phonosurgical technique. Acta Otolaryngol (Stockh) 1974;78:451–7.
45. Strasnick B, Berke GS, Ward PH. Transcutaneous Teflon injection for unilateral vocal cord paralysis: an update. Laryngoscope 1991;101(7 Pt 1):785–7.
46. Arnold GE. Vocal rehabilitation of paralytic dysphonia. I. Cartilage injection into a paralyzed vocal cord. AMA Arch Otolaryngol 1955;62(1):1–17.
47. Dedo HH, Urrea RD, Lawson L. Intracordal injection of Teflon in the treatment of 135 patients with dysphonia. Ann Otol Rhinol Laryngol 1973;82:661–7.
48. Ford CN, Martin DW, Warner TF. Injectable collagen in laryngeal rehabilitation. Laryngoscope 1984;94(4):513–8.
49. Ward PH, Hanson DG, Abemayor E. Transcutaneous Teflon injection of the paralyzed vocal cord: a new technique. Laryngoscope 1985;95(6):644–9.
50. Jako GJ. Laser surgery of the vocal cords. An experimental study with carbon dioxide lasers on dogs. Laryngoscope 1972;82(12):2204–16.
51. Polanyi TG, Bredemeier HC, Davis TW. A CO2 laser for surgical research. Med Biol Eng 1970;8(6):541–8.
52. Strong MS, Jako GJ. Laser surgery in the larynx: early clinical experience with continuous CO_2 laser. Ann Otol Rhinol Laryngol 1972;81:791–8.
53. Strong MS. Laser excision of carcinoma of the larynx. Laryngoscope 1975;85(8): 1286–9.
54. Dumon JF, Reboud E, Garbe L, et al. Treatment of tracheobronchial lesions by laser photoresection. Chest 1981;81:278–84.
55. Anderson RR, Parrish JA. Selective photothermolysis: precise microsurgery by selective absorption of pulsed radiation. Science 1983;220(4596):524–7.
56. Tan OT, Hurwitz RM, Stafford TJ. Pulsed dye laser treatment of recalcitrant verrucae: a preliminary report. Lasers Surg Med 1993;13:127–37.

57. McMillan K, Shapshay SM, McGilligan JA. A 585-nanometer pulsed dye laser treatment of laryngeal papillomas: preliminary report. Laryngoscope 1998; 108(7):968–72.
58. Franco RA Jr, Zeitels SM, Farinelli WA, et al. 585-nm pulsed dye laser treatment of glottal dysplasia. Ann Otol Rhinol Laryngol 2003;112:751–8.
59. Zeitels SM, Akst LM, Burns JA. Office-based 532-nm pulsed KTP laser treatment of glottal papillomatosis and dysplasia. Ann Otol Rhinol Laryngol 2006;115(9): 679–85.
60. Winslow JR. Reports of cases illustrating our progress in the surgical treatment of chronic stenosis of the larynx and trachea. Trans Am Laryngol Assoc 1909;31: 177–90.
61. Jackson C. Stenosis of the larynx with special reference to curative treatment with core molds. Trans Am Laryngol Rhinol Otol Soc 1936;42:12–24.
62. Koempel JA, Cotton RT. History of pediatric laryngotracheal reconstruction. Otolaryngol Clin North Am. 2008;41(5):825–35.
63. Plummer HS. The value of a silk thread as a guide in esophageal technique. Surg Gynecol Obstet 1910;10:519.
64. Hertz AE. Achalasia of the cardia. Quart J Med 1914;8:300–8.
65. Maloney WH. A tapered esophageal bougie. Trans Annu Meet Am Bronchoesophagol Assoc 1960;10.
66. London RL, Trotman BW, DiMarino AJ Jr, et al. Dilatation of severe esophageal strictures by an inflatable balloon catheter. Gastroenterology 1981;80(1):173–5.
67. Rees CJ. In-office unsedated transnasal balloon dilation of the esophagus and trachea. Curr Opin Otolaryngol Head Neck Surg 2007;15(6):401–4.
68. Rees CJ, Fordham T, Belafsky PC. Transnasal balloon dilation of the esophagus. Arch Otolaryngol Head Neck Surg 2009;135(8):781–3.

Anesthesia for Office Procedures

Sean X. Wang, MD, C. Blake Simpson, MD*

KEYWORDS

• Office-based procedures • Laryngeal lesions • Transnasal laryngoscopy
• Flexible laryngoscopy • Tracheoscopy • Topical lidocaine

KEY POINTS

- Most procedures for laryngotracheoesophageal pathologies can be addressed solely through the nose.
- Flexible endoscopy, whether as transnasal esophagoscopy (TNE) or to monitor transoral injection augmentation, is a staple of office-based procedures.
- Typically, diagnostic tracheobronchoscopy only requires 2 mL to 3 mL of topical anesthesia.
- Amide and ester anesthetics reversibly block the sodium channels of the lipid membrane in nerve membranes; these anesthetics are more effective at penetrating unmyelinated nerve fibers that carry autonomic, pain, and temperature impulses.
- Judicious application of topical anesthesia has high safety profile and usually requires minimal patient monitoring.
- The toxicity threshold for anesthesia may be lower for those with systemic medical problems. When in doubt, patient safety may dictate a visit to the operative suite.

BACKGROUND

In the past 20 years, office-based procedures, fueled by advancements in endoscopy technology and pushed by the trend toward minimally invasive procedures, have expanded the armamentarium of many otolaryngologists. These procedures encompass diagnosis and intervention of the larynx, tracheobronchial tree, and esophagus. Technology, skill, and experience of the physician can determine success or failure of an office-based procedure; yet, none of the former can overcome an inadequately anesthetized patient who is uncomfortable and anxious. This article discusses the techniques and pharmacology of anesthesia for office-based procedures.

APPROACHES

The choice of approaches toward achieving adequate anesthesia for office-based procedures is dictated by the experience of the surgeon and the assistant, the

---

Disclosures: The authors have nothing to disclose.
Department of Otolaryngology–Head and Neck Surgery, Medical Arts and Research Center, University of Texas Health and Science Center in San Antonio, Mail Code 8300, 8300 Floyd Curl Drive, San Antonio, TX 78229, USA
* Corresponding author.
E-mail address: SIMPSONC@uthscsa.edu

Otolaryngol Clin N Am 46 (2013) 13–19
http://dx.doi.org/10.1016/j.otc.2012.08.014 **oto.theclinics.com**

selection of equipment, the target location of treatment, the duration of treatment, and patient anatomy/tolerance.

Transnasal Approach

Most procedures for laryngotracheoesophageal pathologies can be addressed solely through the nose, because most otolaryngologists are well trained in flexible laryngoscopy. Before the start of the procedure, both nasal cavities are sprayed with topical 2% oxymetazoline followed by 2% tetracaine. Based on the experience of the senior author (C.B.S.), the most effective way to apply nasal anesthesia is by providing multiple short pulses of spray directed along the floor of the nose. A working channel flexible laryngoscope is then passed transnasally to provide an indirect view of the base of the tongue and laryngopharyngeal complex.

Through the working channel, approximately 1 mL of 4% lidocaine is applied to the base of the tongue, and the remaining 2 mL to 4 mL are applied as 0.5 mL to 1 mL individual aliquots to the laryngeal surface of the epiglottis, supraglottis, and true vocal folds during phonation (holding a long *E*), which produces the "laryngeal gargle," a term coined by Hogikyan.[1] For anesthesia of the tracheobronchial tree, at the end of the phonatory gesture, the patient is instructed to breathe deeply to inspire the lidocaine while being informed that first few breaths will trigger a strong cough reflex. This deep inspiration is usually not needed for procedures isolated to the larynx. The endpoint of adequate anesthesia is marked by the following:

1. Absence of cough reflex during lidocaine aspiration
2. Absence of gag reflex
3. Anesthesia of the larynx during palpation of the epiglottis, base of the tongue, posterior glottis, and bilateral true vocal folds

This approach, if adequately performed, allows procedures of the larynx and tracheobronchial tree. Typically, diagnostic tracheobronchoscopy requires only 2 mL to 3 mL of topical anesthesia.

Transoral Approach

Delivering lidocaine through the mouth is an alternative to the transnasal approach, as initially described by Hogikyan.[1] This approach still requires the video guidance of a flexible laryngoscope. Indications for this approach include surgeon/patient preference or narrow nasal passage that precludes passage of a larger working channel endoscope. The administration of topical anesthesia transorally should be performed in the following sequence:

1. Spray the base of tongue, palate, and posterior pharynx with topical cetacaine spray (13% benzocaine/2% butamben/2% tetracaine).
2. Apply nasal anesthesia (as described previously) to allow insertion of the flexible laryngoscope.
3. Drip 3 mL to 5 mL of 4% lidocaine onto the base of tongue and larynx using an Abraham cannula or a laryngotracheal atomizer spray device (MAD 600, Wolfe Tory Medical, Salt Lake City, Utah) under endoscope guidance.

PATIENT SELECTION

Office-based procedures are well tolerated by most patients. Nevertheless, the following patient characteristics should be considered before embarking on the procedure.

Nasal Patency

Flexible endoscopy, whether as TNE or to monitor transoral injection augmentation, is a staple of office-based procedures. The distal-chip flexible laryngoscope (ENF-VQ, Olympus Surgical, Orangeburg, New York), used in the authors' practice, has an outer diameter of 3.6 mm. The working channel endoscope (ENF-VT2, Olympus, Center Valley, Pennsylvania) has an outer diameter of 4.9 mm. The patient must have a unilateral nasal passage large enough to accommodate the largest endoscope needed for the procedure without significant discomfort.

Oral Passage

For transoral procedures, an interincisor distance of 2 cm or greater is recommended to allow instrumentation.

Gag Reflex

Gag reflex is triggered by the afferent branch of cranial nerve IX. This response varies greatly between individuals. A hyperresponsive gag may be present even with adequate administered topical anesthesia thus rendering flexible endoscopy and/or transoral instrumentation impossible.

Patient Cooperation/Tolerance

Most office-based procedures take 5 to 15 minutes to complete. Procedures, especially those that address the true vocal folds, require patients to remain still and upright. Patients with significant head tremor, vocal fold movement, or torticollis are challenging to treat.

TOPICAL ANESTHESIA SAFETY

Topical or local anesthetics are classified into 2 groups:

1. Amides
2. Esters

These agents consist of an aromatic and an amine group separated by an intermediate group. The class that has an ester link between the intermediate group and the aromatic portion is called esters, and the amides have an amide link.

Examples of esters include

- Tetracaine
- Benzocaine
- Procaine

Examples of amides are

- Lidocaine
- Mepivacaine
- Prilocaine
- Bupivacaine
- Etidocaine

A mnemonic device is that the names of amides contain 2 *i*'s compared with only 1 *i* seen in esters.

When applied topically or locally, amide and ester anesthetics reversibly block the sodium channels of the lipid membrane in nerve membranes. These anesthetics are more effective at penetrating unmyelinated nerve fibers that carry autonomic, pain, and temperature impulses.[2] The main considerations in the clinical use of these agents are potency, duration of anesthesia, the speed of onset, and maximum dose. Potency is determined by the lipid solubility of the agent. Less potent local anesthetics must be given in higher concentration and larger doses. The ability of the anesthetic to bind to proteins in the sodium channel predicts its duration of anesthesia. The onset of action relates to how fast the agent can diffuse through tissues to the nerve. A general reference maximum dose normally exists for various anesthetics; however, actual toxic dose depends on individual patients and their ability to clear the drug.

Lidocaine

Lidocaine has a low to intermediate potency, 45 to 60 minutes duration of action, and onset of sufficient anesthesia within 90 seconds of topical administration. Lidocaine solutions can be found in 1%, 2%, and 4% solutions. The dosage can be calculated from the percentage of lidocaine. For example, 1% lidocaine contains 10 mg/mL, and, for the purpose of office-based procedures, 4% lidocaine translates into 40 mg/mL of lidocaine. Five milliliters of 4% lidocaine equals 200 mg. Commonly quoted maximum dose of 3 mg/kg to 5 mg/kg (pure lidocaine without epinephrine) can lead to systemic toxicity. A 70-kg patient can receive approximately 300 mg of lidocaine. The authors recommend weighing all patients before performing any office-based procedure.

Topical application of lidocaine

Topical application of lidocaine for the purpose of office-based procedures rarely exceeds the toxic dose. Lidocaine-associated toxicity has not been cited in the otolaryngologic literature for the purpose of office-based laryngotracheoesophageal procedures. Postma and colleagues[3] reported 700 consecutive cases of TNE performed in the office using 4% lidocaine without a single case of lidocaine related adverse events (see the article by Bush and Postma elsewhere in this issue). Verma and colleagues[4] published 68 cases of TNEs with 4% topical lidocaine without adverse effects. From the senior author's experience of more than 200 cases of KTP laser treatment of benign vocal fold lesions (Wang, Fuller and Simpson, personal communication, 2011), not a single procedure was aborted due to lidocaine-related adverse effects. The importance of lidocaine's pharmacology and safety profile, however, cannot be overlooked to prevent potential lidocaine toxicity.

Lidocaine toxicity

The half-life of lidocaine is 90 minutes regardless of mode of administration.[5] Systemic reactions to lidocaine involve the central nervous system (CNS) and the cardiovascular system, with the CNS more susceptible. The typical neurologic symptoms of lidocaine toxicity include lightheadedness and dizziness followed by visual and auditory disturbances, such as difficulty focusing and tinnitus. Signs of CNS toxicity are usually excitatory, which may include shivering, muscular twitching, and tremors. Unrecognized and untreated overdose may lead to generalized seizures, followed by coma and respiratory depression.[2] The depressant effects predominate at higher doses. Cardiovascular toxicity of lidocaine derives from the inhibition of sodium channels in the nerve membrane. Lidocaine exerts a dose-dependent negative inotropic effect on cardiac muscle, reducing contractility and interfering with conduction. Lidocaine toxicity can be potentiated by renal impairment, liver disease, and cardiac conditions.

If there is evidence of central nervous system involvement or cardiovascular instability, local anesthetics application and procedure should be discontinued. Pulse oximetry and hemodynamic monitoring should be initiated. Early oxygen supplementation could prevent hypoxia and acidosis and halt progression toward seizure and cardiovascular collapse.[6] When significant overdose is suspected, patients need to be transferred to a facility with anesthesia and ICU support. The detailed management of local anesthetic toxicity is outside the scope of this article. The authors refer to the guidelines published by the American Society of Regional Anesthesia.[6]

Lidocaine allergy

True topical lidocaine allergy during endoscopy has not been reported. There have been reports of lidocaine causing both type I and type IV allergic reactions, however, during dental and cutaneous procedures.[7,8]

Methemoglobinemia from lidocaine

Methemoglobinemia is a rare complication caused by the oxidation of hemoglobin from the ferrous state (Fe^{2+}) to the ferric state (Fe^{3+}). In the ferric state, hemoglobin cannot bind oxygen, thus leading to desaturations. Methemoglobinemia induced by lidocaine has been reported in the bronchoscopy literature when combined with benzocaine, a more powerful oxidizing agent.[9] Methemoglobin is darker than unoxygenated hemoglobin and can produce chocolate cyanosis, a violet or brown discoloration on the lips, ears, and mucous membranes. Systemic symptoms of methemoglobinemia may vary from anxiety to headaches, fatigue, coma, and even death. Methemoglobin levels less than 30% usually resolve spontaneously over 15 to 20 hours when the offending agent is removed and oxygen is administered. For severe cases, methylene blue can be administered at a dose of 1 mg/kg to 2 mg/kg intravenously slowly over 3 to 10 minutes.[9]

Tetracaine

Tetracaine is a highly potent local anesthetic with duration of anesthesia between 60 to 120 minutes when applied topically. According to anesthesiology literature, tetracaine has a slow onset and may take up to 10 minutes to achieve adequate anesthesia[2]; however, based on the authors' experience, it seems to establish the anesthesia of the nasal passage faster than lidocaine. Furthermore, as topical nasal anesthesia, tetracaine has demonstrated superiority to cocaine and lidocaine both in terms of duration of action and pain control.[10–12] Bourolias and colleagues[11] showed that 2% tetracaine solution resulted in significantly less nasal discomfort when compared with 10% lidocaine with transnasal laryngoscopy. Similarly, 2% tetracaine plus adrenaline demonstrated improved intraoperative pain controlled compared with 4% cocaine for septoplasty.[10]

Tetracaine toxicity

Significant tetracaine associated toxicity has not been reported when applied topically through the nose. The half-life and systemic absorption of nasal tetracaine spray have not been clearly defined in the literature. Earlier reports of fatalities with local mucosal application of tetracaine came at doses greater than 100 mg.[13] The authors do not routinely measure the dose of 2% tetracaine nasal spray applied during office-based procedures; however, it is recommended to use less than 1 mL of 2% tetracaine for nasal anesthesia. Typically, only 0.1 mL to 0.2 mL is needed when delivered through an atomizer. The authors do not recommend dripping tetracaine for office-based procedures because this route of application can significantly escalate the dose delivered.

Combining tetracaine and lidocaine

Tetracaine is of ester class of local anesthetics, unlike lidocaine, which is an amide. Animal study has shown that when combining amide and ester anesthetics, their effects are neither synergistic nor antagonistic.[14] This relationship may not hold true in humans, however, and clinicians should be cautioned to not use maximum doses of 2 different local anesthetics, regardless of their class, in combination, assuming that their toxicities are independent.

SAFETY AND MONITORING

As otolaryngologists continue to expand the scope of office-based procedures, patient safety becomes an increasing concern. Most reports in the literature are subjective observation of patient comfort without any hemodynamics monitoring. Postma and colleagues[3] described 700 consecutive cases of TNE performed in the office with minimal complications. Koufman and colleagues[15] reviewed 443 cases of office-based laser procedures with a minor complication rate of 0.9% and no major complications. Rees and colleagues[16] reported high comfort level in 131 patients undergoing office-based pulsed-dye laser treatment.

Manipulation within the laryngotracheoesophageal complex may trigger vasovagal response and lead to nausea, sweating, lightheadedness, and paresthesias before syncope occurs.[15,16] If prodrome of syncope occurs, the procedure should be discontinued, and the patient should assume a reclined or supine position or place the head between the legs with vital signs monitored. If syncope occurs, the patient should remain supine until consciousness is regained.

Given the deficiency of objective data on safety monitoring during office-based procedures, Yung and Courey[17] retrospectively analyzed the hemodynamic changes in patients receiving office-based procedures and noted significant changes in blood pressure and heart rate in 7 of 31 and 9 of 31 patients, respectively. One procedure was terminated due to severe hypertension. A follow-up study performed by the same group prospectively reported the hemodynamic effects of office-based procedures on 50 patients.[18] The data points in this study were recorded at baseline, after the application of nasal decongestant, nasal anesthesia, and insertion of the flexible endoscope. There was a significant change in heart rate after the procedure; furthermore, the placement of the scope in the nasopharynx and hypopharynx was associated with a significant rise in systolic blood pressure and heart rate, respectively. No procedures were prematurely aborted. The investigators concluded that although the hemodynamic changes were apparent, these changes might not be clinically significant. The best advice is to exercise keen clinical judge based on patient anatomy, tolerance, and comorbidities. For patients with known cardiopulmonary disease, performing the procedure in the operative suite should be considered, using appropriate hemodynamic and pulse oximetry monitoring.

POSTPROCEDURE CARE

Patients should be instructed to take nothing by mouth for approximately 60 to 90 minutes after the procedures to prevent aspiration. Globus sensation immediate after the procedure due to anesthesia of the laryngopharyngeal complex is expected. Pain medication is rarely required after office-based procedures; if needed, acetaminophen usually suffices.

SUMMARY

With the acceleration of today's medical technology, otolaryngologists continue to push the limits of office-based procedures. As new frontiers in the realms of laryngotracheoesophageal complex are explored, efficacious and safe application of topical anesthetics is a prerequisite. Topical lidocaine in the laryngopharynx and nasal application of tetracaine can provide adequate anesthesia for majority of the office-based procedures, but the potential complications associated with these local anesthetics must be clearly understood and anticipated. The toxicity threshold may be lower for those with systemic medical problems. Whenever in doubt, patient safety may dictate a visit to the operative suite.

REFERENCES

1. Hogikyan ND. Transnasal endoscopic examination of the subglottis and trachea using topical anesthesia in the otolaryngology clinic. Laryngoscope 1999;109(7 Pt 1):1170–3.
2. Berde CB, Strichartz GR. Local anesthetics. In: Miller RD, Eriksson LI, Fleisher LA, et al, editors. Miller's anesthesia. 7th edition. Philadephia (PA): Churchill, Livingstone Elsevier; 2009:913–40.
3. Postma GN, Cohen JT, Belafsky PC, et al. Transnasal esophagoscopy: revisited (over 700 consecutive cases). Laryngoscope 2005;115:321–3.
4. Verma SP, Smith ME, Dailey SH. Transnasal tracheoscopy. Laryngoscope 2012; 122(6):1326–30.
5. McCaughey W. Adverse effects of local anaesthetics. Drug Saf 1992;7:178–89.
6. Neal JM, Bernards CM, Butterworth JF 4th, et al. ASRA practice advisory on local anesthetic systemic toxicity. Reg Anesth Pain Med 2010;35(2):152–61.
7. Chiu CY, Lin TY, Hsia SH, et al. Systemic anaphylaxis following local lidocaine administration during a dental procedure. Pediatr Emerg Care 2004;20(3): 178–80.
8. Kaufmann JM, Hale EK, Ashinoff RA, et al. Cutaneous lidocaine allergy confirmd by patch testing. J Drugs Dermatol 2002;2:192–4.
9. Kwok S, Fischer JL, Rogers JD. Benzocaine and lidocaine induced methemoglobinemia after bronchoscopy: a case report. J Med Case Rep 2008;2:16.
10. Drivas EI, Hajiioannou JK, Lachanas VA, et al. Cocaine versus tetracaine in septoplasty: a prospective, randomized, controlled trial. J Laryngol Otol 2007;121(2): 130–3.
11. Bourolias C, Gkotsis A, Kontaxakis A, et al. Lidocaine spray vs tetracaine solution for transnasal fiber-optic laryngoscopy. Am J Otolaryngol 2010;31(2):114–6.
12. Noorily AD, Otto RA, Noorily SH. Intranasal anesthetic effects of lidocaine and tetracaine compared. Otolaryngol Head Neck Surg 1995;113(4):370–4.
13. Adriani J, Campbell D. Fatalities following topical application of local anaesthetics to mucous membranes. JAMA 1956;162:1527–30.
14. Liu PL, Feldman HS, Giasi R, et al. Comparative CNS toxicity of lidocaine, etidocaine, bupivacaine, and tetracaine in awake dogs following rapid intravenous administration. Anesth Analg 1983;62(4):375–9.
15. Koufman JA, Rees CJ, Frazier WD, et al. Office-based laryngeal laser surgery: a review of 443 cases using three wavelengths. Otolaryngol Head Neck Surg 2007;137:146–51.
16. Rees CJ, Halum SL, Wijewickrama RC, et al. Patient tolerance of in-office pulsed dye laser treatments to the upper aerodigestive tract. Otolaryngol Head Neck Surg 2006;134:1023–7.
17. Yung KC, Courey MS. The effect of office-based flexible endoscopic surgery on hemodynamic stability. Laryngoscope 2010;120:2231–6.
18. Ongkasuwan J, Yung KC, Courey MS. The physiologic impact of transnasal flexible endoscopy. Laryngoscope 2012;122(6):1331–4.

Laryngoscopy, Stroboscopy and Other Tools for the Evaluation of Voice Disorders

Lucian Sulica, MD

KEYWORDS

• Stroboscopy • Diagnosis • Hoarseness • Dysphonia

KEY POINTS

- Evaluation of voice disorders consists of the history, including a characterization of individual vocal demand and behavioral elements contributing to the voice disorder, perceptual assessment of the voice, and laryngoscopy.
- Dysphonia results from disruptions of phonatory physiology. To be most effective, diagnostic evaluation of dysphonia must focus on dynamic assessment of laryngeal function.
- Stroboscopy is the only technique that allows routine clinical imaging of vocal fold oscillation, and as a result is likely the single strongest diagnostic instrument in most cases of dysphonia.
- A discrepancy between the preliminary diagnostic impressions based in history and acoustic assessment and laryngoscopic findings is a warning that the evaluation is not complete. Rather than embarking in empiric treatment of poorly defined diagnoses, further, more refined imaging techniques must be used to resolve the discrepancy.

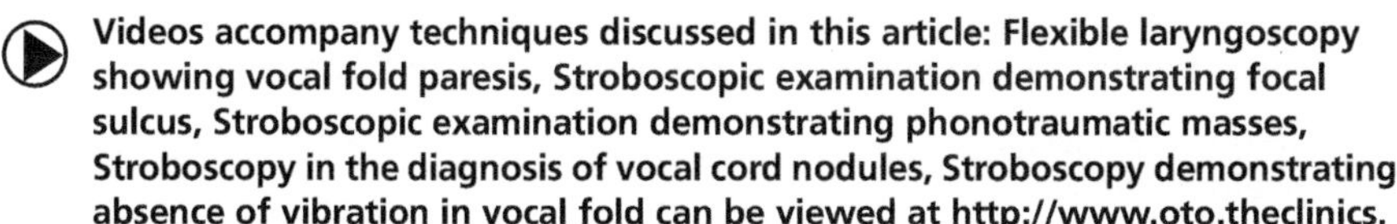

Videos accompany techniques discussed in this article: Flexible laryngoscopy showing vocal fold paresis, Stroboscopic examination demonstrating focal sulcus, Stroboscopic examination demonstrating phonotraumatic masses, Stroboscopy in the diagnosis of vocal cord nodules, Stroboscopy demonstrating absence of vibration in vocal fold can be viewed at http://www.oto.theclinics.

The diagnostic evaluation of voice disorders has always been an office-based undertaking. Its central task is visualization of the larynx, without which no definitive diagnosis may be made. Steady progress in laryngeal visualization has allowed ever more refined diagnoses to be made. However, quality differences in laryngoscopy have been largely ignored in the otolaryngology literature, which typically treats all types of office examination as if they were equal. In fact, examination quality has

Laryngology/Voice Disorders, Department of Otolaryngology-Head & Neck Surgery, Weill Cornell Medical College, 1305 York Avenue, 5th Floor, New York, NY 10021, USA
E-mail address: lus2005@med.cornell.edu

Otolaryngol Clin N Am 46 (2013) 21–30
http://dx.doi.org/10.1016/j.otc.2012.09.001 oto.theclinics.com
0030-6665/13/$ – see front matter

tremendous clinical impact in an area where functional disturbances can be caused by small or subtle abnormalities.

Although key, laryngeal visualization is also only a part of a broad and thoughtful approach to the complaint. A brief overview of the scope of such an evaluation before consideration of aspects of laryngoscopy is useful.

EVALUATION OF VOICE DISORDERS

Hoarseness is the colloquial term for dysphonia; both terms are often used interchangeably in medicine to refer to altered voice quality. Hoarseness may be both a symptom and a sign of dysfunction of the phonatory apparatus. It is never a diagnosis, despite having a corresponding ICD code and sometimes serving as such for purposes of administrative convenience. The breadth of pathology that can cause hoarseness makes a unified overview a challenge; hoarseness is simply not a homogenous category after the first laryngoscopy. Nevertheless, certain unifying principles exist.

History

Voice disorders have resisted straightforward objective clinical characterization, despite the array of instrumental measures of acoustics and aerodynamics available. In most cases, important personal and subjective considerations influence the voice complaint, as well the patient's treatment expectations. As a consequence, medical evaluation of voice disorders requires attention to several factors not encompassed by the usual history solicited from patients with head and neck complaints. These include careful characterization of the complaint, both with respect to its nature and its severity, and an assessment of the patient's voice demands and habits. This approach emphasizes the functional limitations caused by the patient's voice problems.

Through history taking, the otolaryngologist must first understand for what aspects of impaired voice production the patient seeks help. Patient perceptions of voice problems tend to be individual and directly connected with the amount and type of vocal demands; for example, a school teacher's notion of "hoarseness" is likely to differ substantially from a singer's or a construction foreman's. The word "hoarseness" is used broadly to describe a variety of phenomena, and can refer to:

- Altered voice quality;
- Phonatory fatigue;
- Insufficient loudness;
- Restricted pitch range;
- Increased phonatory effort;
- Breathlessness;
- Impaired singing quality; and
- Other features.

It is not always the feature most obvious to the clinician which the patient finds troublesome.

The perception of the severity of these complaints is also subject to personal interpretation. Individuals have expectations and requirements of their voices that are not always a direct reflection of their occupational demands or other easily assessed factor, and often different from what the otolaryngologist might assume. Many people with dysphonia never seek medical attention, unaware that any problem exists. Others simply want to be reassured that their dysphonia is not caused by a malignancy. Still others complain of phonatory disturbances that are not apparent to the casual listener, and can even consider these crippling to professional or social activity. In part to help characterize the severity of an individual's voice problem, several standardized and statistically validated questionnaires have been developed. Among them, the Voice Handicap Index[1] and the Voice-Related Quality of Life[2] are the most widely used. The Voice Handicap Index-10[3] is an abridgment of the former that makes it even easier to use without loss of statistical validity. Such inventories are useful to understand patient motivation and make appropriate treatment recommendations. Applied both before and after treatment, these can also form an important means of assessing outcome, which allows comparison among interventions, techniques, and studies.

Phonotrauma refers to the physical stress on the tissues of the vocal fold during phonation. It is considerable and has the potential to cause changes to the oscillatory properties of the vocal folds and local tissue injury.[4,5] Because phonotrauma may be the single most important factor underlying most benign vocal fold lesions, assessing its extent and severity is an essential task of the voice history. Independent of medical factors, phonotrauma is related to amount and intensity of voice use, which in turn may be the product of vocal demand. Vocal demand usually results from an individual's professional requirements, and inappropriate or excessive voicing, usually owing to an inherently talkative and extroverted personality. Distinguishing between demand and personal inclination is important to making appropriate treatment recommendations. The term "vocal abuse" has been used broadly and somewhat indiscriminately as a synonym for phonotrauma. However, it is not always correct, and almost never helpful, simply to blame the patient for his vocal predicament. Teachers, for example, are notoriously overrepresented among voice patients, owing largely to the relentless vocal demand of their work rather than any intrinsic behavioral factors.

Examination

The voice examination too has specialized elements, not least among them the use of the ear as a diagnostic instrument. Qualitative assessment of the voice precedes laryngoscopy. Gross abnormalities are readily apparent to the ear as the patient describes the complaint; more subtle ones require specific maneuvers and phonatory tasks to search for breakdowns of phonatory physiology. Low-intensity, high-pitched phonation which results in voice breaks, irregularities, and delays in voice onset suggests a small mucosal lesion. Reduced maximum phonation time (normally >20 seconds) and limitations in volume point to poor glottic closure. Phonation of a sustained vowel may be required to clearly reveal a tremor or other instability; connected speech or other complex task may be necessary to identify dysfluency such as laryngeal dystonia.

Based on the contents of the history and the voice assessment, the clinician should develop a diagnostic impression before visualization of the larynx. It is generally possible to assign a particular case to a category—mucosal disturbance, glottic insufficiency, or neurologic movement disorder—before laryngoscopy. Discrepancy between this preliminary impression and subsequent findings should serve as warning that the evaluation is not complete. A flexible fiberoptic examination that reveals no mucosal pathology when voice qualities suggest that it must be present is not a rare clinical situation. Rather than settling on a vague and nonspecific diagnosis—"chronic laryngitis" and "reflux" are the current favorites—the physician should progress to rigid endoscopy, stroboscopy, and even more specialized techniques to resolve the discrepancy.

The well-known GRBAS scale,[6] and more recently, the CAPE-V,[7] represent efforts to systematize qualitative voice assessment and standardize the terminology used. These serve a descriptive rather than a diagnostic purpose. Although not essential for routine clinical practice, they are useful to focus the assessment and for inquiry into clinical outcomes and efficacy.

LARYNGOSCOPY

Office evaluation concerns itself with indirect laryngoscopy, that is, the transmission of the image of the larynx to the examiner through the medium of an optical instrument. Because this allows observations while the patient is awake and reasonably comfortable, it is possible to perform a functional assessment of the larynx, a key distinction from the more anatomic emphasis of the rest of the traditional head and neck examination. An appreciation of function is essential in an area of otolaryngology that concerns itself with restoration of normal physiology more than excision of pathology.

Larynx Visualization

The larynx may be visualized by mirror, rigid peroral endoscope, and flexible transnasal endoscope. The instrument should be distinguished from the optical technique. In particular, rigid peroral endoscopy has often been conflated with stroboscopy because, historically, flexible fiberoptic endoscopy offered inadequate image quality for stroboscopic examination. The venerable laryngeal mirror has the advantage of crisp optical resolution and color fidelity but, in practice, these do not offset the inability to record the examination and the occasional technical difficulty of the examination.

Flexible Laryngoscope

The flexible laryngoscope in its fiberoptic version is available in nearly every otolaryngologist's office and offers the surest means of visualizing the vocal folds. Rarely, patients find the examination intolerable. Flexible laryngoscopy also disturbs normal laryngeal dynamics least, permitting laryngeal visualization during connected speech, a feature that makes the flexible laryngoscope the instrument of choice for the evaluation of most neurologic disorders. The typical findings of spasmodic dysphonia, tremor and other diseases may change or disappear when the patient is maneuvered into a nonphysiologic position for peroral laryngoscopy. Similarly, glottic dynamics in cases of vocal fold paralysis or paresis may be more reliably evaluated without tongue traction (**Fig. 1**, Video 1). However, because of dependence of optic fibers, the flexible fiberoptic scope is optically inferior to every other means of examining the larynx,

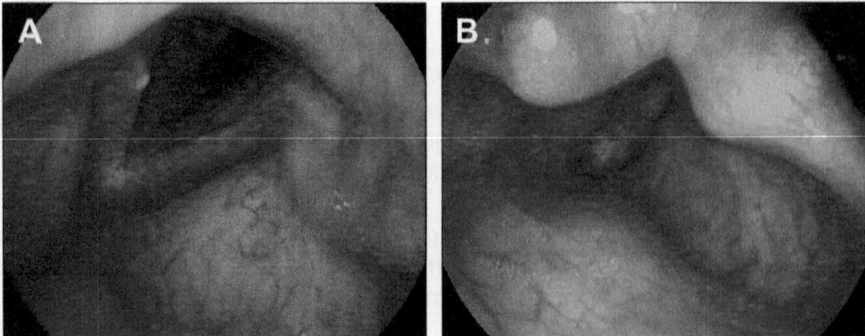

Fig. 1. 66 year old man with left sided vocal fold paresis. During respiration (1a), note thinning and atrophy of the left vocal fold. During phonation (1b), note hyperfunction of contralateral (neurologically intact) ventricular fold.

including the mirror, and does not reliably reveal small mucosal lesions. New designs that convert the optical signal to digital information at the tip of the endoscope (so-called chip tip devices) do away with fibers and improve the picture.

Rigid Endoscope

The rigid endoscope, which transmits the image to the eyepiece via a glass rod, offers high-resolution optical qualities at the price of increased technical skill, similar to that required to handle a laryngeal mirror. As a result, it is a superior mean of evaluating mass lesions and mucosal abnormalities.

Depth Perception

The limited depth perception offered by all commonly used techniques of office examination tends to obscure the 3-dimensional nature of laryngeal function. Efforts to extrapolate this from careful examination have not always proved reliable and may lead to significant diagnostic confusion. The endoscopist should always keep this limitation in mind.

Stroboscopy

So far, we have been speaking exclusively of continuous light examination. Stroboscopy uses a pulsed light source to create an illusion of continuous, slow-motion mucosal oscillation. The light pulses at a frequency just slightly different from that of the glottal cycle, generating a series of still images of the vocal fold at slightly different points across several glottal cycles that are then fused into an apparently fluid and continuous sequence by the examiner's eye. Video 2 The stroboscopic effect depends on appropriate timing of the light pulses in relation to phonatory frequency, and so is most reliable when vocal fold oscillation is periodic. Aperiodicity of mucosal vibration is often an important component of dysphonia. If severe, it tends to compromise stroboscopic light timing and thus the quality of the examination. Despite this limitation, stroboscopy is the only practical way of imaging mucosal oscillation routinely in the clinic, and the optimal—and occasionally the only—way of identifying abnormalities in mucosal pliability. It is likely the single strongest diagnostic instrument in most cases of dysphonia, especially for those disorders related to disturbances of mucosal vibration (eg, scar and sulcus) (**Fig. 2**, Video 3). Stroboscopy is traditionally performed via rigid instrumentation but the improved optics of distal chip flexible laryngoscopes have made flexible stroboscopy both practical and useful.

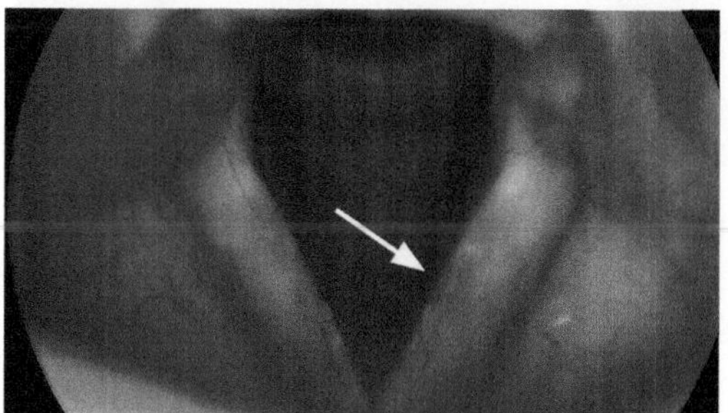

Fig. 2. The excellent optics of the rigid endoscope and stroboscopic light are key in identifying a focal sulcus of the left vocal fold which has an important impact on this performer's voice.

The utility of stroboscopy is increased by video recording, important not only for documentation, but also to enhance the accuracy of the examination. Review, both at normal and reduced speeds, can reveal aspects of pathology not seen on the initial examination, even if it is meticulous and unhurried. Video recording is essential for comparison across time and accurate and revealing assessments of clinical interventions (**Figs. 3** and **4**, Videos 4 and 5).

The role of stroboscopy in the evaluation of hoarseness has not been precisely established, but its diagnostic power has been underrepresented in the literature. Strobolaryngoscopy is especially likely to be helpful whenever the findings of laryngoscopic examination under continuous light do not explain the severity of the patient's complaint, when hoarseness persists despite the treatment of its supposed cause, and when there is unexpected hoarseness after microlaryngoscopy.[8–10]

Some unusual mucosal abnormalities, such as sulcus and mucosal bridges, remain difficult to discern even with stroboscopy, although the alteration in mucosal wave pliability should draw the surgeon's attention to the affected area. Stroboscopy should not be relied upon to determine the presence or absence of invasion in epithelial mucosal lesions and does not replace biopsy in these cases (**Fig. 5**, Video 6).

Most diagnostic errors probably result from failing to resolve a discrepancy between the preliminary diagnostic impressions and laryngoscopic findings. A flexible fiberoptic examination that reveals no mucosal pathology when voice qualities suggest that it must be present is a rare clinical situation. Such a scenario should serve as warning that the evaluation is not complete. In this context, empiric treatment of vague and nonspecific diagnoses, such as "postnasal drip," "chronic laryngitis," and "reflux" instead of proceeding to rigid endoscopy, stroboscopy, and even more specialized techniques is likely to yield only delay in diagnosis. Reflux is particularly problematic, because this diagnosis is often made from suggestive findings on laryngoscopy which are neither sensitive nor specific, prompt improvement is not expected, and the literature supports progressive increase in medication dosage in the absence of response. Together, these may result in months-long diagnostic delays. In fact, reflux is very rarely—if ever—the primary cause of a complaint of hoarseness, although it may be an aggravating secondary factor.

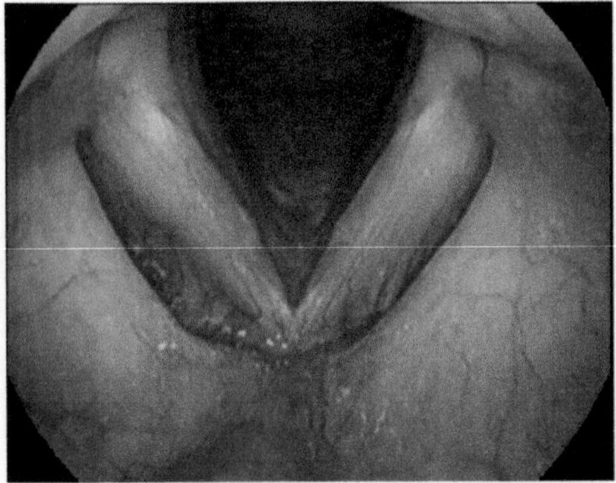

Fig. 3. Stroboscopy via a flexible laryngoscope is used to diagnosed midfold phonotraumatic masses in this 23 year old voice student, a common pathology. Compare with **Fig. 4** & Video 5 below.

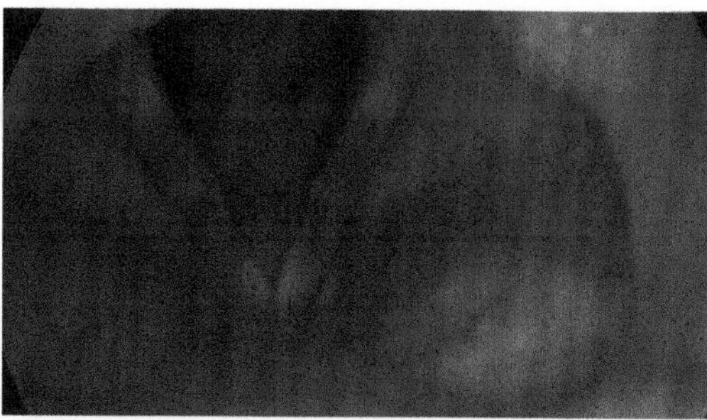

Fig. 4. Stroboscopy helps in the accurate diagnosis of rheumatoid nodules of the vocal folds, so called "bamboo nodes," in this 26 year old woman with ill-defined connective tissue disease. Note that these cause far more disturbance to mucosal wave vibration than ordinary phonotraumatic masses shown in **Fig. 3**.

INVESTIGATIONAL TECHNIQUES

High-Speed Cinematography

High-speed cinematography has recently become available for office use, although it remains expensive. High-speed filming developed concurrently with xenon light technology, and was initially designed to study jet engine performance. It was adapted to visualize laryngeal vibration during the middle of the 20th century, but its clinical value in the study of laryngeal vibratory function remains unknown. Therefore, the technology has yet to be widely applied in clinical practice, a situation that may change as companies commercialize the technology and investigators explore its potential.

In high-speed cinematography, between 2000 and 6000 separate images are captured each second. This is the first imaging technology with a capture rate faster than vocal fold vibration. This allows the evaluation of vocal fold vibration without the problem of missing aspects of the vocal fold vibratory activity, particularly when vibrations are aperiodic. Because stroboscopy depends on aliasing, or producing a representation of vibration from a montage of images across multiple vibratory cycles, it is particularly blind to the latter situation, as discussed. Original high-speed

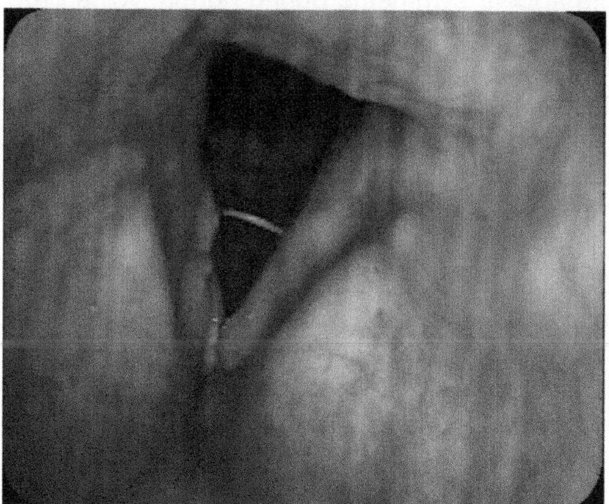

Fig. 5. The absence of vibration in the right vocal fold is extremely concerning in this 67 year old attorney. While this cannot be relied upon to demonstrate invasion, it is a highly suggestive finding. At biopsy, the lesion proved to be squamous cell carcinoma.

cinematography units actually used 35-mm film exposed with a xenon arc lamp so rapidly that after exposure, the film had to be allowed to roll out onto the floor. Video technology now allows images to be captured and digitized for instant playback. The few commercially available units allow the user to select the rate of image capture. At present only rigid peroral rod-lens technology transfers light from the xenon light source efficiently enough to allow adequate resolution.

The obvious advantage of the higher capture rate is greater detail in mucosal movement during phonation. The disadvantage is that the sheer amount of data requires a substantial amount of time to analyze. If we assume that most video technology plays images back at rate of 30 frames per second, then viewing 4000 frames captured in 1 second of voice production requires over 2 minutes at the standard playback rate. Commercially available units allow the examiner to choose 2-second segments of voice production to image. Practically, it is often difficult to determine which 2 seconds of voicing are clinically important and then equally challenging to analyze those 2 seconds. Several researchers have focused on vibratory patterns at onset of phonation, in vocal folds with lesions and after periods of extended voice use.[11–13] These studies, although well done, have not yet yielded information that has impacted clinical practice. In contrast, even though stroboscopy only provides a representation of mucosal vibration, it does allow/encourage extended observation across multiple pitches and intensities. From this information, clinicians have been able to identify altered vibratory patterns associated with clinically relevant disease states. However, because we learn more with clinical study, we may find that high-speed cinematography provides useful data at certain points during voice production, such as vocal onset or offset, so that the information achieves clinical relevance.

Kymography

Kymography is an outgrowth of high-speed cinematography with video capture. In kymography, the examiner selects 1 horizontal plane (essentially 1 raster line of the video image) of the glottis for detailed visualization. The vibratory motion of the vocal fold in that plane, as it moves toward and away from the midline, is then plotted in the vertical axis. This allows the examiner to study the movement of the most medial aspect of the vocal fold toward and away from the midline. In this manner, if the endoscope is oriented exactly perpendicular to the axis of the glottis, the movement of the medial edges should appear symmetric during normal voice production. In patients with altered voice, vocal fold edges may be plotted to move asymmetrically or at different speeds.[14] As with any examination technique, there are many variables, ranging from the placement of the endoscope to choosing the correct plane of vibration for study and the correct voice segment. With further study, videokymographic observations may help to improve our ability to diagnose altered laryngeal vibratory patterns.[15]

Narrow Band Imaging

Narrow band imaging (NBI) visualizes the larynx using selected portions of the light spectrum, or "narrow bands." Visible light, perceived as white light, is energy from the electromagnetic spectrum of wavelengths between 400 and 700 nm. Different wavelengths are perceived as different colors. The shorter wave lengths are blue in hue and the longer wavelengths are red. Color is perceived from the wavelength that is reflected back from the object. For example, an apple appears red because the surface absorbs the blue/green wavelengths and reflects back the red. As light encounters tissue, it is absorbed and scattered. The long wavelengths (red) diffuse deeply, whereas the shorter wavelengths (blue) diffuse more superficially. Because some cancers arise in the superficial epithelium of tissue and are associated with the abnormal proliferation of blood vessels owing to angiogenesis, NBI technologies select only the shorter wavelengths of light to view tissue.[16] By filtering light to limit it to bands in the 400- (blue spectrum) and 540-nm (green spectrum) range, which are preferentially absorbed by the hemoglobin pigment in the superficial vasculature, abnormal superficial blood vessels can be made to seem dark and thus more obvious to the examiner.[17] In esophageal cancer, NBI imaging is being studied to determine whether routine surveillance can pick up these abnormal vascular patterns before they can be identified with standard visible light endoscopy. Similar studies are being performed for cancers in the head and neck area.[18,19] For cancers not associated with keratosis, NBI screening may provide an advantage over standard endoscopy for early detection. In lesions that are keratinized, such as many laryngeal lesions, the technology may be less useful as keratosis reflects all of the visible light and seems white.

SUMMARY

Hoarseness is both a sign and a symptom of dysfunction of the phonatory apparatus, and can be the product of a number of disorders. Accurate diagnosis of the cause via the history and examination is the essential task in the hoarse patient. Timely and thorough laryngoscopy is the core diagnostic test. This is achievable with an array of readily available technologies. Continuous light sources, such halogen light, can be paired with standard flexible endoscopic technology to examine the larynx and hypopharynx during a wide variety of physiologic tasks. Optimal high-resolution inspection of the vocal folds proper may be achieved via rigid peroral rod-lens endoscopes. Although there has been debate regarding the optimum technique, the argument is an artificial one, because both rigid and flexible endoscopy may easily be performed in the same patient if there is a need.

In cases in which detailed examination of vocal fold mucosa and its vibratory characteristic are indicated, particularly those in which the cause of the hoarseness is not clear on continuous light laryngoscopy, stroboscopic examination may be undertaken using either rigid or flexible instrumentation. The best combination of light carriers and image transmission for this examination technique remain the rigid peroral rod-lens endoscopes, but rigid instruments should in no way be considered the only means by which stroboscopic examination may be performed. Using modern distal chip technology, stroboscopic images of a quality approaching those of rigid rod-lens instruments may be obtained via flexible endoscopes.

At this writing, high-speed cinematography, kymography, and NBI remain experimental means of imaging laryngeal and hypopharyngeal anatomy and function.

Modern laryngology, and particularly laryngeal surgery, has become a functional endeavor. The aim of treatment is no longer simply to excise pathology, but rather to restore the normal physiology of phonation. For this to succeed, the otolaryngologist must understand phonatory anatomy and physiology, the utility of the diagnostic tools available, the range of possible problems and the patient's own vocal demands and expectations.

SUPPLEMENTARY DATA

Supplementary data related to this article can be found online at http://dx.doi.org/10.1016/j.otc.2012.09.001.

REFERENCES

1. Jacobson GA, Johnson A, Grywalski C, et al. The Voice Handicap Index (VHI): developemnt and validation. Am J Speech Lang Pathol 1997;6:66–70.
2. Hogikyan ND, Sethuraman G. Validation of an instrument to measure voice-related quality of life. J Voice 1999;13:557–69.
3. Rosen CA, Lee AS, Osborne J, et al. Development and validation of the voice handicap index-10. Laryngoscope 2004;114:1549–56.
4. Gray SD, Hammond E, Hanson DF. Benign pathologic responses in the larynx. Ann Otol Rhinol Laryngol 1995;104(1):13–8.
5. Dikkers FG. Nodules, polyps, reinke edema, metabolic deposits and foreign body granulomas. In: Fried MP, Ferlito A, editors. The larynx. 3rd edition. San Diego (CA): Plural; 2009. p. 181–90.
6. Imaizumi S. Acoustic measure of roughness in pathological voice. J Phonetics 1986;14:457–62.
7. American Speech-Language-Hearing Association special interest division 3, voice and voice disorders. Consensus auditory perceptual evaluation of voice (CAPE-V). 2003. Available at: http://www.asha.org. Accessed July 1, 2012.
8. Casiano RR, Zaveri V, Lundy DS. Efficacy of videostroboscopy in the diagnosis of voice disorders. Otolaryngol Head Neck Surg 1992;107(1):95–100.
9. Sataloff RT, Spiegel JR, Hawkshaw MJ. Strobovideolaryngoscopy: results and clinical value. Ann Otol Rhinol Laryngol 1991;100(9 Pt 1):725–7.
10. Woo P, Casper J, Colton R, et al. Diagnosis and treatment of persistent dysphonia after laryngeal surgery: a retrospective analysis of 62 patients. Laryngoscope 1994;104(9):1084–91.
11. Patel R, Dailey S, Bless D. Comparison of high-speed digital imaging with stroboscopy for laryngeal imaging of glottal disorders. Ann Otol Rhinol Laryngol 2008; 117:413–24.
12. Mendelsohn AH, Sung MW, Berke GS, et al. Strobokymographic and videostroboscopic analysis of vocal fold motion in unilatereal superior laryngeal nerve paralysis. Ann Otol Rhinol Laryngol 2007;116:85–91.
13. Kunduk M, Yan Y, McWhorter AJ, et al. Investigation of voice initiation and voice offset characteristics with high speed digital imaging. Logoped Phoniatr Vocol 2006;31:139–44.
14. Qiu Q, Schutte HK. A new generation videokymography for routine clinical vocal fold examination. Laryngoscope 2006;116:1824–8.
15. Svec JG, Sram F, Schutte HK. Videokymography in voice disorders: what to look for. Ann Otol Rhinol Laryngol 2007;116:172–80.
16. Muto M, Katada C, Sano Y, et al. Narrow band imaging: a new diagnostic approach to visualize angiogenesis in superficial neoplasia. Clin Gastroenterol Hepatol 2005;3(7 Suppl 1):S16–20.
17. Kuraoka K, Hoshino E, Tsuchida T, et al. Early esophageal cancer can be detected by screening endoscopy assisted with narrow-band imaging. Hepatogastroenterology 2009;56:63–6.
18. Masaki T, Katada C, Nakayama M, et al. Narrow band imaging in the diagnosis of intra-epithelial and invasive laryngeal squamous cell carcinoma: a preliminary report of two cases. Auris Nasus Larynx 2009;36(6):712–6.
19. Orita Y, Kawabata K, Mitani H, et al. Can narrow band imaging be used to determine the surgical margin of superficial hypopharyngeal carcinoma? Acta Med Okayama 2008;62:205–8.

In-office Evaluation of Swallowing

FEES, Pharyngeal Squeeze Maneuver, and FEESST

Albert L. Merati, MD

KEYWORDS

- Dysphagia • Swallowing • Flexible endoscopic evaluation of swallowing
- Flexible endoscopic evaluation of swallowing sensory testing • Laryngoscopy
- Pharynx

KEY POINTS

- In-office evaluation of dysphagia is a fundamental part of caring for patients with swallowing complaints. Patients with dysphagia must undergo examination of the main organs of swallowing: larynx, pharynx, and tongue.
- Although flexible fiber optic laryngoscopy itself is a powerful tool in assessing patients with swallowing difficulties, the addition of a few simple steps allows for FEES, a well-studied, simple, and intuitive test of swallowing function.
- Clinical evaluation of pharyngeal motor strength can be accomplished with the pharyngeal squeeze maneuver; this is performed in a matter of seconds during flexible fiber optic laryngoscopy and has a strong correlation with more involved and more invasive measures.
- FEESST includes *S*ensory *T*esting with the FEES component. Despite promising early studies, FEESST has not become a common or widely used tool in the evaluation of swallowing dysfunction.
- The presence of *bilateral* deficits as determined by FEESST is a powerful clinical indicator of poor swallowing.

OVERVIEW

Dysphagia contributes to the dominant causes of morbidity and mortality in patients cared for by otolaryngologists,[1–3] including the leading cause of death in this group—aspiration pneumonia complicating stroke. The overall morbidity and medical complexity of these cases and the perceived lack of opportunities for surgical intervention many contribute to reluctance and even disinterest among some otolaryngologists in the detailed evaluation of patients with swallowing disorders. It is the rare

Division of Laryngology, Department of Otolaryngology – HNS, University of Washington School of Medicine, Box 356515, 1959 Northeast Pacific, Seattle, WA 98195, USA
E-mail address: amerati@uw.edu

Otolaryngol Clin N Am 46 (2013) 31–39
http://dx.doi.org/10.1016/j.otc.2012.08.015
oto.theclinics.com
0030-6665/13/$ – see front matter

dysphagia patient seen in the outpatient setting that will undergo surgery for that problem.[4] Nonetheless, important decisions must be made with regard to the feeding status, diet, and airway safety of these patients. Even patients without overt swallowing complaints should, depending on their overall clinical scenario, undergo the simple tests characterized in this article. One common example of this is in patients with unilateral vocal fold paralysis. Although predominantly thought of as a voice problem, many of these patients have swallowing problems as well. Heitmiller and colleagues[5] recently reported on modified barium swallow studies performed on patients with known unilateral vocal fold paralysis. In this report, 38% of the studies found aspiration with 12% finding laryngeal penetration, a significant fraction in any group. This emphasizes the value of evaluating swallowing function in all laryngology consultations.

No group of physicians is more appropriate or capable of caring for this often-challenging group than otolaryngologists; improving and mastering the in-office evaluation of dysphagia patients begins with knowledge and familiarity with the flexible endoscopic evaluation of swallowing (FEES) examination and the pharyngeal squeeze maneuver. Flexible endoscopic evaluation of swallowing sensory testing (FEESST) is also discussed an attractive but less commonly used adjunct.

Flexible Endoscopic Evaluation of Swallowing

The intuitive and embraceable nature of the FEES examination has been a key part of its attraction for clinicians evaluating dysphagic patients. What could be more fundamental than literally looking into the pharynx and larynx during swallowing and noting what happens with material presented to the patient to swallow? The FEES examination was introduced in 1988 by Langmore and colleagues[6] in the journal *Dysphagia*.

Patient preparation and positioning

The FEES procedure is ideally done with the patient in the seated position, unreclined, and totally awake. Sometimes these important examinations are performed at the bedside for inpatients at acute or chronic care facilities where patients cannot sit up. If possible, the most ideal condition for safe oral intake (position, wakefulness) is reproduced for FEES testing. One of the many advantages that FEES testing has over the modified barium swallow (MBS) is the ability to obtain useful clinical information without transporting patients (often infirm, unstable, or needing to travel a great distance) to a hospital with MBS facilities.

Although most studies cited in this section advocate (and even insist) that no local anesthesia be applied topically to the nose, as is customary for other flexible fiber optic laryngoscopy (FFL) examinations, opinion on this does vary. The concern driving this proscription is that the presence of anesthetic sprayed in and through the nasal cavity may alter pharyngeal or laryngeal function.

In one study of healthy young controls, Rubin and colleagues[7] were not able to identify any obvious motion abnormalities in patients before versus after the administration of topical anesthetic for FFL. This study was helpful, but without larger numbers and a study group that included patients with laryngeal and pharyngeal dysfunction, it is difficult to say that the presence of topical anesthesia is innocuous.

Recently, a large Cochrane Review was performed looking not at the possible impact of topicalization on function but rather on its utility and necessity in anesthetizing the nose for FFL in the first place. The authors found no compelling evidence supporting its use.[8] Predictably, the lack of strong evidence one way or another was lacking. Finally, Suiter and Moorhead[9] executed a helpful study examining the impact of the presence of a fiber optic scope in the pharynx (transnasally placed) on MBS findings. In a study of 14 normal subjects, ranging from ages 23–83 years, the presence of an FFL past the soft palate but above the epiglottis did not affect swallow duration, bolus clearance, or penetration/aspiration scale (PAS) scores. This finding helps of course, with concerns over the observer effect of FEES on swallowing function. This study has not been reproduced in a population of symptomatic patients.

Aging effects on penetration/aspiration

FEES is capable of discriminating changes that occur with age even in an asymptomatic population. Butler and colleagues[10] studied a series of young adults and compared them with a similarly sized group of subjects with a mean age of 75 years. The PAS score was significantly different between the 2 groups, who also had longer dwell times and more residue. Butler and colleagues[11] follow this up with a prospective study of a group of 76 older subjects (age 60 years and older) with no swallowing complaints; their group specifically looked at liquid type, bolus size, and delivery method (straw vs cup) in this investigation. Penetration was found in up to 83% of subjects, and aspiration was seen in 24% of those studied. It should be noted that this took many swallows in some cases to detect these events. Nonetheless, they did occur. The PAS scores were clearly worse with milk versus water swallows, larger volumes, and straw use. These findings should be considered in the interpretation of FEES examinations on dysphagic clinic patients.

What is the role of the FEES examination? FEES is good at detecting the presence of penetration, aspiration, pooling, retained secretions, and the effectiveness of coughing in a given patient. It is also good at detecting even small amounts of material passing superiorly into the nasopharynx during swallowing.

FEES technique

- The FEES begins with the patient in the seated position.
- If a videostroboscopy is indicated for other reasons, it should be performed first.
- Once the patient and team (often an otolaryngologist and a speech language pathologist) are ready, the pharyngeal squeeze maneuver is performed first.
- The oral intake challenges begin with water or ice chips.

Some clinics, such as the University of Washington Laryngology Program, use some food coloring to help with the identification of retained food or liquid; this method is useful for training purposes and also for patients and their families. The study itself does not require contrasting colors; Leder and colleagues[12] showed nicely it is not necessary for most FEES examinations. This important study also found remarkable intra- and interrater reliability for FEES.

- If a patient does well with the ice chips or water, pureed consistencies and crackers or pretzels can be administered. Although caution is important in evaluating these patients, a reasonable challenge to their swallowing should be presented in this monitored, idealized setting.
- The presence of penetration or aspiration should be noted.
- Important details should also include noting any vallecular, pharyngeal wall, or pyriform residue.
- As in an MBS, the presence of an expert speech language pathologist (SLP) allows for the implementation of positioning strategies and compensation maneuvers such as head tuck and chin tuck to one side to assess the impact, if any, on swallowing efficiency and safety.[13]

FEES is limited in assessing oral phase problems, although early spillage is easily detected. The MBS is superior to FEES in this regard. The MBS is also better at allowing for quantification of pharyngeal movement, including base of tongue and constrictor activity. The FEES is also limited in terms of describing upper esophageal sphincter (UES) segment transit. Nonetheless, it is an important and valuable adjunct to the clinical evaluation of patients with dysphagia. It requires no more tools than what are already present in most otolaryngologists' offices. It adds little time and minimal discomfort to the patient's evaluation. The FEES may be the only meaningful swallow evaluation available to a remote or difficult-to-move patient.

Pharyngeal Squeeze Maneuver

The pharyngeal squeeze maneuver (PSM) is basic: during FFL, the patient is asked to make high-pitched, strained phonation, preferably in a rising crescendo of effort. This will, in normal pharynges, result in obvious recruitment of the pharyngeal constrictor musculature. It is not a subtle finding.

This simple observation, first characterized and published by Bastian in 1991,[14] has proven to be a useful adjunct to the in-office evaluation of dysphagia patients. What is potent about the PSM is the clinical information it provides in just a few seconds, with zero risk to the patient.

Specifically, Bastian,[14] followed by many others, advocates that the following step is performed during FFL. At a point in the examination before any challenges (FEESST or FEES), "while maintaining a panoramic view, patients are asked to produce the highest pitch of which they are capable." This is meaningful even in the presence of severe dysphonia, ie, it is not the sound produced that matters, it is the recruitment of the pharyngeal musculature.

What can we conclude about the PSM? What does it mean?

Investigators have proposed that its presence endoscopically serves as a reasonable surrogate for the formal testing of pharyngeal motor strength. The University of California Davis group has published extensively on this subject; one of the more important articles from this team compared the endoscopic PSM with the pharyngeal constriction ratio (PCR), a validated measure of pharyngeal strength as seen on contrast fluoroscopy.[15]

PCR correlation with pharyngeal strength

The PCR had been shown previously to inversely correlate with pharyngeal strength, ie, low strength was associated with a higher PCR and vice versa When using the PCR as a reliable indicator of pharyngeal strength, the PSM was also found to be good. The average PCR for dysphagic patients was found to be 0.06 (low number reflecting a good PCR and, by inference, good motor strength in the pharynx), whereas the mean PCR for those dysphagic patients with an absent PSM was 0.31, a statistically significant difference from the PSM-positive group.[16]

PSM as predictor of swallowing safety

Advocates have studied the utility of PSM (focusing on the assessment of pharyngeal motor function) compared with the information obtainable in studying pharyngeal and laryngeal sensory function. In a small but important series of clinical investigations, pharyngeal strength, as inferred from the PSM, serves as an important predictor of swallowing safety—perhaps even more so than tests of sensory function.

PSM qualitative realiability

The PSM has high interrater reliability when the test is treated as qualitative and as a simple question of present or absent. In an article from 2007, Rodriguez and colleagues[17] studied a convenience sample of 40 patients undergoing FFL with

PSM. When the reviewers were asked to categorize the findings for PSM as absent, diminished, or normal, there was weak interrater reliability. When the reviewers simply grouped the studies by normal or abnormal PSM, the reliability was high. Also, the laterality of the test is not reliably assessable (Peter Belafsky, personal communication, 2012).

Food textures in PSM

Specific textures have been studied in terms of the role of PSM in swallowing evaluation. Perlman reported an interesting prospective study of pureed food intake in 204 dysphagic patients.[18] These patients underwent both FEES and sensory testing (FEESST, see later discussion). The patients were divided into groups with normal, moderate, or severe sensory deficits based on their sensory testing. They were also categorized by the presence or absence of the pharyngeal squeeze. One striking finding was that patients did not show an increasing level of aspiration for pureed textures despite increasing levels of sensory disturbance. The authors concluded "the aspiration of pureed foods may depend more on muscle tone of the hypopharynx than on sensation."[18]

Another part of that study looked at similar questions with thin liquid challenges instead of purees. Setzen and colleagues[19] published this study of 204 patients presented with 5-mL liquid boluses during FEES testing. Again, these patients also underwent sensory testing. In the thin liquid study, only 2% of the normal sensation/normal squeeze aspirated. This number increased to 29% with motor function impairment. Patients with a moderate decrease in sensation did not aspirate during their trials as long as motor function, as measured by the presence of a positive PSM, was intact. When the patients with moderate sensory impairment also had any motor impairment, most of them aspirated. Most strikingly, the rate of aspiration in patients with severe sensory impairment but intact motor function was 15% (5 of 33 patients); this increased to 100% (15 of 15) in patients with the same severe level of sensory impairment but a poor pharyngeal squeeze.

PSM related to Zenker's diverticulum

Anecdotally, the author thinks that the presence of a positive PSM is important in counseling patients with Zenker's diverticulum as to their swallowing outcomes postoperatively. Those with intact PSM are more likely to have immediate swallowing success in contrast to those who have already worn out the pharynx or have become malnourished. The presence of a weak pharynx and or significant bilateral pooling in a preoperative patient with Zenker's diverticulum is an indication for a preoperative gastrostomy tube in many cases of Zenker's diverticulum with advanced age or comorbidities.

Flexible Endoscopic Evaluation of Swallowing with Sensory Testing

Investigators have long searched for a minimally invasive, clinically feasible, reliable method to test laryngeal sensory function. Recent advances have included "SELSAP" (Surface-Evoked Laryngeal Sensory Action Potential)[20] in which external, noninvasive electrodes are used to assess superior laryngeal nerve conduction as an indicator of laryngeal sensory function. Until this or other approaches are more refined, the current leading method in the measurement of laryngeal sensory function is the FEESST. Despite a valuable series of supporting articles and studies, FEESST continues to be of modest clinical utility to laryngologists and to otolaryngologists in general.

The fundamental concept driving the FEESST study is that stimulation of the supraglottic larynx, in this case by a small puff of air delivered in close proximity to the laryngeal mucosa, results in elicitation of the laryngeal adductor reflex (LAR).[21] The LAR results in a brisk and easily identifiable closure response to stimulus. The response is noted for both the right and left side; the tests are quantified at various levels of air-puff pressure stimulation.

One typical scenario is to test patients at 3 mmHg on each side and determine the presence or absence of the LAR response. If an LAR is detected, it is noted as normal for this side. Further precision beyond the presence of eliciting an LAR at 3 mmHg is not clinically useful. If no LAR is seen at 3 mmHg, the stimulus is increased to 6 mmHg and retested. If this increase elicits a response, a mild impairment is noted. If no response is elicited at 6 mmHg, the air puff stimulus is set to 9 mmHg. Positive LAR at this level (in the absence of positivity less than this threshold) is recorded as a moderate impairment. No response to stimulus at 9 mmHg is documented as a severe sensory deficit. Both sides are tested. It should be emphasized that the presence of bilateral deficits as determined by FEESST is a powerful clinical indicator of poor swallowing.

Jonathan Aviv, MD, is a main driver of investigation and dissemination of information regarding FEESST. He and others have carefully and comprehensively categorized its safety as an in-office examination.[22,23] Aviv's impact can be readily discerned from this article's reference list. His 2005 book, coauthored with Tom Murry, PhD, is also helpful as a compendium of knowledge and experience regarding FEESST.[24]

The fundamentals of FEESST depend on measuring the presence or absence of the LAR after unilateral stimulation of the supraglottic mucosa by a discreet puff of air, in this case, as delivered through the channel in or alongside a flexible fiber optic laryngoscope. Both sides are tested for the elicitation threshold. The pressure of the air puff can be altered, and the lowest level at which the LAR is seen is noted; the higher air pressure needed, the more impairment of laryngeal sensory function.

One of Aviv's early studies compared psychophysical testing (ie, asking the patient if they can feel the stimulus in the larynx/pharynx) with the FEESST's dependence on the simple LAR.[25] In this elegant study, 20 normal subjects and 80 dysphagic patients were scrutinized and found to have a remarkable correlation between the psychophysical testing and the FEESST, providing solid evidence that the FEESST was an excellent surrogate and, more importantly, could perhaps be used in patients who were not able to participate in the test from a behavioral standpoint.

FEESST in bedridden or incapacitated patients

The ability for FEESST to assess laryngeal and pharyngeal function in the absence of patient participation has been touted as a significant advantage in bedridden or otherwise incapacitated patients. Although this is true, only a fraction of these patients are likely to be safely swallowing. The presence of severe, particularly bilateral, defects in sensation are thought to be indicators for poor swallowing safety. As discussed in the FEES section, clinicians have expressed concern with the possible impact of nasal topical anesthesia on FEESST findings. Johnson and colleagues[26] looked at this in an important study from 2003 in which 15 subjects underwent FEESST with and without topical decongestion and anesthesia; no difference was noted in stimulation thresholds. Once again, however, this study was done in normal volunteers, not in dysphagic patients.

Aviv and colleagues,[27] through an important series of articles, established early that normal subjects had predictable LAR responses to air-puff stimulation. In a study of 20 healthy patients with a mean age of 34 and no symptoms related to swallowing, sensory thresholds for LAR elicitation were consistent (2.9 mmHg

± 0.7). Another study nicely established that laryngeal sensory function, as tested during FEESST, declines with age.[28] In a test of 80 adults across a wide variety of ages:

- The mean threshold for eliciting the LAR was 2.60 mmHg
- For the 20- to 40-year-old subjects, the level was 2.06 mmHg
- For the 41- to 60-year-old group, the level was 2.44 mmHg
- In the subjects older than 60, the level was 2.97 mmHg

The older control group was not at threshold level for sensory deficit, but the trend with time was clearly shown.

FEESST in acute neurologic patients

Perhaps the strongest argument for the utility of the FEESST study is in acute neurologic patients. Aviv and colleagues,[3] in 1997, studied a series of 20 patients who underwent both MBS and FEESST testing in the acute period after stroke. These patients were followed up prospectively for 2 years. Four of the 10 patients with no evidence of aspiration on initial MBS had pneumonia in the follow-up period; most of these patients had significant bilateral deficits on FEESST examination. Of the 5 patients who had no aspiration on MBS and also did not have sensory deficits on FEESST, none had pneumonia during the follow-up period. The authors advocated the use of FEESST as an "adjunct to MBS in guiding the dietary management of stroke patients with dysphagia." In my opinion, these patients are different than many of the complex dysphagia patients that might be seen in a laryngologist or otolaryngologists' office; the OTO patients are more likely to have mucosal damage or inflammation, be it from reflux, radiation, or other form of injury. In my experience, this makes performance and interpretation of FEESST less predictable and, in my hands, less reliable. In patients without significant changes to the surface of the larynx/pharynx, FEESST remains an attractive idea. Aviv,[28] Murry and colleagues,[29] and others have investigated FEESST as a modality to test patients with chronic cough and paradoxic vocal fold dysfunction.[30] The utility of FEESST in characterizing underlying neuropathy in the presence of varying amounts of laryngeal inflammation remains an open question.

SUMMARY

The in-office comprehensive assessment of both simple and complex cases involving laryngeal or pharyngeal dysfunction can be quickly, safely, and meaningfully advanced with the performance of the FEES examination, including assessment of the pharyngeal squeeze maneuver. Although the MBS continues to be the gold standard for the evaluation of swallowing complaints, there is little if any downside to the FEES examination. All dysphagia patients should undergo FFL examination of laryngeal and pharyngeal anatomy and function. While this is being performed, the PSM task and the video documentation of the dedicated FEES examination should be executed whenever possible. Many have argued that these tests do not preclude the use of the MBS—particularly if the patient may have issues related to upper esophageal sphincter dysfunction—an area that the FEES is not as good at detecting. I would argue that the additional time and effort when the patient is already undergoing an FFL, with little if any additional risk to the patient (beyond that which would be incurred with the intake of food or liquid during an MBS) is valuable and may help save the patient a trip to the radiology suite for the MBS on occasion.

REFERENCES

1. Link DT, Willging JP, Miller CK, et al. Pediatric laryngopharyngeal sensory testing during flexible endoscopic evaluation of swallowing: feasible and correlative. Ann Otol Rhinol Laryngol 2000;109(10 Pt 1):899–905.
2. Sitton M, Arvedson J, Visotcky A, et al. Fiberoptic Endoscopic Evaluation of Swallowing in children: feeding outcomes related to diagnostic groups and endoscopic findings. Int J Pediatr Otorhinolaryngol 2011;75(8):1024–31.
3. Aviv JE, Sacco RL, Mohr JP, et al. Laryngopharyngeal sensory testing with modified barium swallow as predictors of aspiration pneumonia after stroke. Laryngoscope 1997;107(9):1254–60.
4. Merati AL, Pawar S. "Surgery for swallowing disorders and aspiration." Textbook of laryngology. San Diego (CA): Plural Publishing; 2007.
5. Heitmiller RF, Tseng E, Jones B. Prevalence of aspiration and laryngeal penetration in patients with unilateral vocal fold motion impairment. Dysphagia 2000; 15(4):184–7.
6. Langmore SE, Schatz K, Olsen N. Fiberoptic endoscopic evaluation of swallowing safety: a new procedure. Dysphagia 1988;2:216–9.
7. Rubin AD, Shah A, Moyer CA, et al. The effect of topical anesthesia on vocal fold motion. J Voice 2009;23(1):128–31.
8. Sunkaraneni VS, Jones SE. Topical anaesthetic or vasoconstrictor preparations for flexible fibre-optic nasal pharyngoscopy and laryngoscopy. Cochrane Database Syst Rev 2011;(3):CD005606.
9. Suiter DM, Moorhead MK. Effects of flexible fiberoptic endoscopy on pharyngeal swallow physiology. Otolaryngol Head Neck Surg 2007;137(6):956–8.
10. Butler SG, Stuart A, Kemp S. Flexible endoscopic evaluation of swallowing in healthy young and older adults. Ann Otol Rhinol Laryngol 2009;118(2):99–106.
11. Butler SG, Stuart A, Leng X, et al. Factors influencing aspiration during swallowing in healthy older adults. Laryngoscope 2010;120(11):2147–52.
12. Leder SB, Acton LM, Lisitano HL, et al. Fiberoptic endoscopic evaluation of swallowing (FEES) with and without blue-dyed food. Dysphagia 2005;20(2):157–62.
13. Rees CJ. Flexible endoscopic evaluation of swallowing with sensory testing. Curr Opin Otolaryngol Head Neck Surg 2006;14(6):425–30.
14. Bastian RW. Videoendoscopic evaluation of patients with dysphagia: an adjunct to the modified barium swallow. Otolaryngol Head Neck Surg 1991;104(3): 339–50.
15. Leonard R, Belafsky PC, Rees CJ. Relationship between fluoroscopic and manometric measures of pharyngeal constriction: the pharyngeal constriction ratio. Ann Otol Rhinol Laryngol 2006;115(12):897–901.
16. Fuller SC, Leonard R, Aminpour S, et al. Validation of the pharyngeal squeeze maneuver. Otolaryngol Head Neck Surg 2009;140(3):391–4.
17. Rodriguez KH, Roth CR, Rees CJ, et al. Reliability of the pharyngeal squeeze maneuver. Ann Otol Rhinol Laryngol 2007;116(6):399–401.
18. Perlman PW, Cohen MA, Setzen M, et al. The risk of aspiration of pureed food as determined by flexible endoscopic evaluation of swallowing with sensory testing. Otolaryngol Head Neck Surg 2004;130(1):80–3.
19. Setzen M, Cohen MA, Perlman PW, et al. The association between laryngopharyngeal sensory deficits, pharyngeal motor function, and the prevalence of aspiration with thin liquids. Otolaryngol Head Neck Surg 2003;128(1):99–102.
20. Bock JM, Blumin JH, Toohill RJ, et al. A new noninvasive method for determination of laryngeal sensory function. Laryngoscope 2011;121(1):158–63.

21. Aviv JE, Martin JH, Keen MS, et al. Air pulse quantification of supraglottic and pharyngeal sensation: a new technique. Ann Otol Rhinol Laryngol 1993;102(10): 777–80.
22. Aviv JE, Murry T, Zschommler A, et al. Flexible endoscopic evaluation of swallowing with sensory testing: patient characteristics and analysis of safety in 1,340 consecutive examinations. Ann Otol Rhinol Laryngol 2005;114(3):173–6.
23. Cohen MA, Setzen M, Perlman PW, et al. The safety of flexible endoscopic evaluation of swallowing with sensory testing in an outpatient otolaryngology setting. Laryngoscope 2003;113(1):21–4.
24. Aviv JE, Murry T. FEESST: flexible endoscopic evaluation of swallowing with sensory testing. San Diego (CA): Plural Publishing; 2005.
25. Aviv JE, Martin JH, Kim T, et al. Laryngopharyngeal sensory discrimination testing and the laryngeal adductor reflex. Ann Otol Rhinol Laryngol 1999;108(8):725–30.
26. Johnson PE, Belafsky PC, Postma GN. Topical nasal anesthesia and laryngopharyngeal sensory testing: a prospective, double-blind crossover study. Ann Otol Rhinol Laryngol 2003;112(1):14–6.
27. Aviv JE, Kim T, Thomson JE, et al. Fiberoptic endoscopic evaluation of swallowing with sensory testing (FEESST) in healthy controls. Dysphagia 1998;13(2):87–92.
28. Aviv JE. Effects of aging on sensitivity of the pharyngeal and supraglottic areas. Am J Med 1997;103(5A):74S–6S.
29. Murry T, Branski RC, Yu K, et al. Laryngeal sensory deficits in patients with chronic cough and paradoxical vocal fold movement disorder. Laryngoscope 2010;120(8):1576–81.
30. Cukier-Blaj S, Bewley A, Aviv JE, et al. Paradoxical vocal fold motion: a sensory-motor laryngeal disorder. Laryngoscope 2008;118(2):367–70.

Transnasal Esophagoscopy

Carrie M. Bush, MD[a,*], Gregory N. Postma, MD[b]

KEYWORDS

• Esophagoscopy • Esophageal sphincter • Transnasal • Surgical procedure

KEY POINTS

- Transnasal esophagoscopy (TNE) is performed in the office setting and obviates the need for sedation.
- TNE has been found to be both safe and efficacious. Its diagnostic accuracy is equal to sedated conventional endoscopy.
- The ability to perform TNE in awake patients decreases the cost and increases the safety of the procedure compared with conventional sedated esophagoscopy.
- TNE is valuable for both esophageal screening, as well as multiple in office procedures (ie, tracheoesophageal puncture, esophageal dilation, biopsy).
- As TNE becomes more common, the indications and role for the procedure will become more defined.

Video of transnasal esophagoscopy in-office procedure accompanies this article at http://www.oto.theclinics.com/

Otolaryngologists are frequently consulted to assist in management of patients requiring esophagoscopy for a thorough evaluation of their symptoms.[1–3] The diagnostic applications of transnasal esophagoscopy (TNE) have now become widespread. Patients with history of dysphagia, globus, extraesophageal reflux and gastroesophageal reflux disease are often well managed by the otolaryngologist without requiring further referral to a gastroenterologist. With TNE, the otolaryngologist may examine from the nasal cavity to the level of the gastroesophageal junction (GEJ) and cardia of the stomach. Biopsies and additional procedures may be performed as needed. Furthermore, the ease and safety of TNE has made it invaluable, particularly in the care of patients with medical comorbidities and head and neck cancer.

[a] Department of Otolaryngology, Georgia Health Sciences University, 1120 15th Street, Augusta, GA 30912, USA; [b] Department of Otolaryngology, Center for Voice, Airway and Swallowing Disorders, Georgia Health Sciences University, 1120 15th Street, Augusta, GA 30912, USA

* Corresponding author.

E-mail address: cabush@georgiahealth.edu

Otolaryngol Clin N Am 46 (2013) 41–52
http://dx.doi.org/10.1016/j.otc.2012.08.016
oto.theclinics.com

TNE in Comparison to Conventional Endoscopy

As with most new technology, TNE was originally met with skepticism. Some early studies showed a lack of promise with concern generated in regard to the efficacy of the procedure. However, with increased user familiarity and further technological advancement, TNE has risen in popularity. Recent studies are uniformly in agreement that TNE has diagnostic capabilities that are equal to that of conventional endoscopy (CE). In a study by Jobe and colleagues,[4] there was noted to be a good degree of agreement between TNE and CE on both endoscopic and histologic findings. Other studies have concluded that TNE biopsies are accurate, with a 97% congruence to those of CE.[5] There is a high degree of correlation between TNE and CE, with TNE being 89% sensitive and 97% specific.[3] Of interest, TNE has also been associated with higher patient satisfaction rates when compared with CE.[6–9]

The great promise in TNE is that it may be performed without sedation. Sedation is responsible for the majority of adverse events (>50%) associated with CE,[10] such as aspiration, oversedation, hypoventilation, vasovagal episodes, and airway obstruction. In a 2007 national survey of endoscopists, sedation was found accountable for 67% of complications and 72% of mortality associated with CE.[11] These adverse events are all eliminated by the performance of unsedated esophagoscopy.

The ability to perform TNE awake also significantly decreases the cost of the procedure in comparison with CE. Direct costs, such as longer procedure time, recovery time, medications, and monitoring and nursing expenses are accrued with sedation. Indirect costs, such as loss of work, and need for a caretaker and driver are associated with sedation. Recent studies have estimated as much as a $2000 per-procedure cost savings with TNE versus CE.[12]

Indications

Although the role of TNE continues to define itself with time and user experience, the current indications are broad and may be divided into 3 categories (**Table 1**): (1) Esophageal, (2) extra-esophageal, and (3)Procedure related. By permitting direct visualization of the esophagus, TNE may be used to diagnose esophagitis, strictures, rings, hiatal hernias, webs, neoplasms, vascular anomalies, and diverticula. The tone of the lower esophageal sphincter may be assessed; high tone may be indicative of achalasia or pseudoachalasia. In addition, subjective peristaltic activity may be determined by assessing passage of liquids and solids during the examination. (Liquids should transit the esophagus within 13 seconds.)

Table 1
Indications for TNE May Be Divided into 3 Main Categories

Esophageal	Extra-Esophageal	Procedure Related
Dysphagia	Significant globus	Pan-endoscopy for head and neck cancer
Refractory gastroesophageal reflux disease	Screening for head and neck cancer	Biopsy
Abnormal imaging	Moderate to severe EER	Botox injection
Screening for Barrett's	Chronic cough	Balloon dilation
		Percutaneous endoscopic gastrostomy
		Tracheoesophageal puncture
		Placement of wireless pH monitoring device

Other applications for TNE are being evaluated

***Helicobacter pylori* infection** TNE may be used to document resolution of *H pylori* infection. In patients with cirrhosis or after liver transplantation at high risk for post-sedation encephalopathy, TNE serves as an ideal alternative to detect and grade esophageal varices.[13] Patients who require frequent screening (history of head and neck cancer or caustic ingestion) also serve to benefit from the safety and ease of TNE. In morbidly obese patients at high risk with sedation, TNE is now commonly being performed before bariatric surgery[14] and to evaluate the postoperative gastrointestinal tract as well.

Nasopharyngeal stenosis and neopharyngeal stricture TNE has been proven successful for a number of in-office procedures. Hydrostatic balloons may be used to dilate narrow segments of the esophagus, as well as treat post-radiation nasopharyngeal stenosis and neopharyngeal stricture after total laryngectomy. Laser fibers may be advanced through the TNE working channel for treatment of recurrent respiratory papillomas and tumors. Secondary tracheoesophageal puncture can be performed on the awake patient. Percutaneous endoscopic gastrostomy may be performed; Botox can be injected into muscles of the esophagus[15]; feeding tubes can be inserted, and wireless pH monitoring devices may be placed as well.[16]

Foreign bodies There is limited application of TNE in management of foreign bodies (FB). Patients may be screened for esophageal FB,[6] with definitive management in cases in which the FB may be pushed into the stomach. However, should retrieval be required TNE is not recommended as the airway may be placed at risk.

Barrett's esophagus The use of TNE for screening of Barrett's esophagus has gained many advocates. In the past 30 years, esophageal adenocarcinoma has become the most rapidly increasing neoplasia in the United States.[17,18] Barrett's esophagus is recognized as a premalignant lesion, with 0.5% of patients developing malignant transformation each year.[19] Symptoms of extraesophageal reflux, including chronic cough, are known to be more predictive of esophageal adenocarcinoma than symptoms of classic gastroesophageal reflux disease.[20] Given the cost and morbidity associated with conventional esophagoscopy, current guidelines suggest empiric treatment of gastroesophageal reflux disease and extraesophageal reflux before esophagoscopy. As the use of TNE continues to evolve, guidelines may change to recommend earlier esophagoscopy. However, once diagnosed, surveillance of Barrett's esophagus is performed with CE to allow for comfortable completion of a full, 4-quadrant set of biopsies spaced every 2 cm of Barrett's esophagus with large biopsy instruments.

Head and neck cancer TNE is emerging as an invaluable instrument for management of head and neck cancer patients. Initial panendoscopy may be performed in the office setting, and esophageal screening may be performed on a routine basis. In previous studies, TNE has been shown to provide 100% accuracy in biopsy results and staging of tumor when compared with standard panendoscopy.[21] By obviating the need for sedation and operating room facilities, TNE decreases the time, costs, and risks involved with standard panendoscopy. TNE screening in head and neck cancer patients after treatment has also proved worthwhile. In a group of head and neck cancer patients undergoing TNE, only 13% were found to have normal examinations. Pathology ranged in severity, and included peptic esophagitis, stricture, candidiasis, Barrett's metaplasia, gastritis, and carcinoma.[22] Screening with TNE in head and neck cancer patients has revealed a 4% to 5% rate of metachronous esophageal cancer, with a significantly higher prevalence (15.9%) in patients with a history of hypopharyngeal cancer.[22,23] The most appropriate protocol to use after head and neck cancer patients with TNE is not known at this time.

Contraindications

There are no absolute contraindications to TNE. The presence of diverticula may make TNE more difficult to perform. Although some have questioned TNE in anticoagulated patients, it is the experience of the senior author and others that both examination and biopsy may be performed without complication in patients on clopidogrel (Plavix) or Warfarin (Coumadin).

PREOPERATIVE PLANNING

Before the procedure, one should become familiar with the equipment. There are a number of venders through which a transnasal esophagoscope may be obtained (EE-1580 K, Pentax Precision Instrument Corporation, Orangeburg, New York; Olympus PEF-V, Olympus America Inc, Melville, New York; and; Viscion Sciences TNE-2000 with Endosheath, Medtronic Xomed, Jacksonville, Florida). Transnasal esophagoscopes are generally 60 cm longer to allow adequate length for visualization of the stomach and retroflexion. They vary in width from 3.1 to 5.1 mm (compared with 10–12 mm for the conventional esophagoscope) and have capacity for suction, irrigation, and insufflation. A working channel is present though which instruments (biopsy forceps, laser fibers, and channels for topical anesthesia application) may be introduced.

Patients should be asked to remain NPO at least 3 hours before the procedure. This decreases the risk of regurgitation and aspiration. However, recent oral intake is not an absolute contraindication to TNE.

PATIENT PREPARATION AND POSITIONING

The patient in placed in the otolaryngology office examination chair in the sitting position. As routine, vital signs are obtained. However, continuous monitoring of vital signs throughout the procedure is not necessary. Although this may be appropriate for elderly individuals with severe hypertension or coronary artery disease. Appropriate nasal anesthesia and decongestion is essential for tolerance of the procedure. A 1:1 solution of oxymetazalone 0.05% and lidocaine 4% is aerosolized and applied topically to the nasal cavity. The solution is then applied to a cotton pledget and the nasal cavity is packed for 10 minutes. A spray of 20% benzocaine (Hurricaine) may be administered to the oropharynx. Viscous lidocaine is used by some examiners. Although anesthesia is essential, excess anesthesia has potential to increase the difficulty of the procedure. Should the hypopharynx become overly anesthetized secretions will pool, leading to aspiration and subsequent coughing during the procedure.

PROCEDURAL APPROACH

See Video of TNE in-office procedure that accompanies this article.

- The endoscope is lubricated and introduced into the nasal cavity and preferably passed along the nasal floor to the nasopharynx. Depending on patient anatomy, the endoscope may need to be introduced between the middle and inferior turbinates.

- The endoscope is then advanced beyond the nasopharynx to allow for visualization of the larynx and hypopharyx.
- The patient is asked to flex their head and the endoscope is held in position just superior to the post-cricoid region.
- The patient is then asked to swallow to allow for gentle introduction of the transnasal esophagoscope into the esophagus.
- Air insufflation and suction are used as needed to carefully and rapidly advance the instrument (with lumen in sight at all times) beyond the lower esophageal sphincter to the stomach.
- Retroflexion is then performed to allow a view of the endoscope passing through the GEJ and cardia of the stomach. This is performed by rotating the entire endoscope 180° and maximally deflecting the endoscope tip 210°. Extra air is often required to allow for adequate visualization.
- At completion of this portion of the procedure, the additional air is suctioned from the stomach to prevent patient discomfort.
- The endoscope is then slowly withdrawn and the distal esophagus is carefully evaluated with particular care taken in the examination of the GEJ.
- The remainder of the esophagus is meticulously examined with use of air insufflation, suction, and irrigation to allow for best visualization of the esophageal mucosa.
- Biopsy forceps are passed through the working channel if needed to sample esophageal lesions.

Anatomic Considerations

Given the small size of the transnasal endoscope, the view will differ from that of rigid or CE. The small size of the scope is less likely to distort the natural anatomy, and external compressions and natural curvature may be more prominent.[24] There are 3 major curves in the esophagus.

1. The most proximal occurs at the base of the neck as the esophagus veers left then returns to midline at T5.
2. At T7 there is a second gentle left curve.
3. At the distal esophagus there is a slight anterior curve as the esophagus passes through the diaphragm.

There are also 3 areas of external compression:

1. Most proximally is that of the aorta, which may be visualized as a pulsating mass at the left anterolateral wall of the esophagus (**Fig. 1**).
2. The left mainstem bronchus may be observed as an anterior compression 2 cm beyond the level of the aorta (**Fig. 2**).
3. At the distal aspect of the esophagus the diaphragm will be viewed as a circumferential compression (**Fig. 3**), which becomes more prominent when the patient is asked to "sniff."

Evaluation of the distal esophagus is a key portion of TNE. Suspicion for a hiatal hernia may be raised when there seems to be a loose diaphragmatic crus on retroflexion. By definition, if gastric rugae extend more than 2 cm above the diaphragm, a hiatal hernia is present. The squamocolumnar junction or meeting of the esophageal and gastric mucosa, should naturally occur at the GEJ or junction of the gastric rugae and network of terminal esophageal vessels. On appearance, the squamous epithelium tends to have a gray-white hue, whereas the gastric mucosa is salmon pink

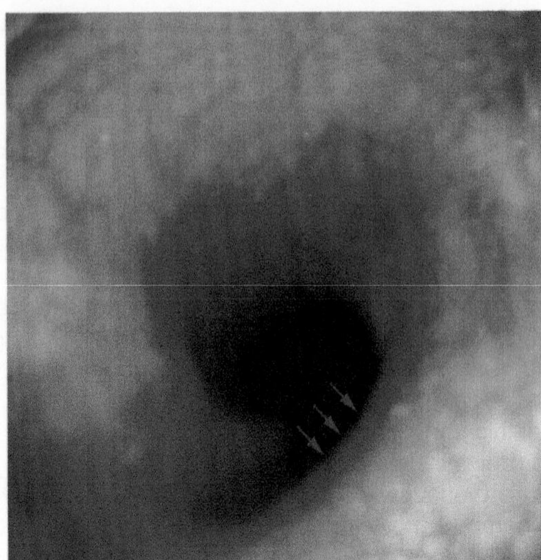

Fig. 1. The aorta may be visualized as a pulsating mass at the left anterolateral wall of the esophagus.

(**Fig. 4**). If the squamocolumnar junction is proximal to the GEJ, this is evidence of clinical Barrett's esophagus, and biopsies should be performed.

IMMEDIATE POSTPROCEDURE CARE

One of the great benefits of TNE is that no postprocedure care is required. The patient is asked to remain sitting in the examination chair for several minutes before departure. They are then returned to the ambulatory setting, free to drive themselves home or to work at their discretion.

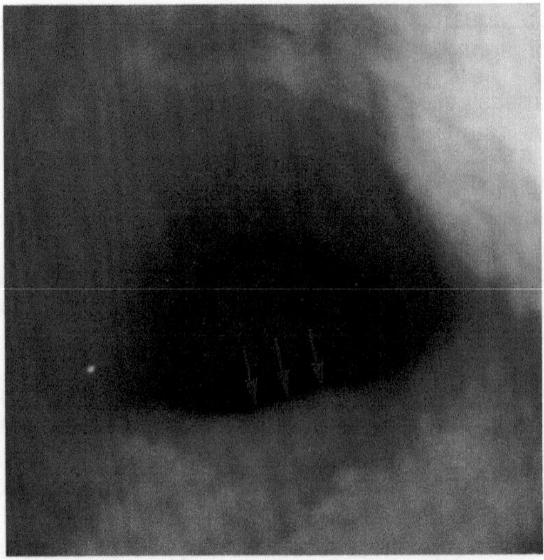

Fig. 2. The left mainstem bronchus compresses the esophagus 2 cm distal to the aortic arch.

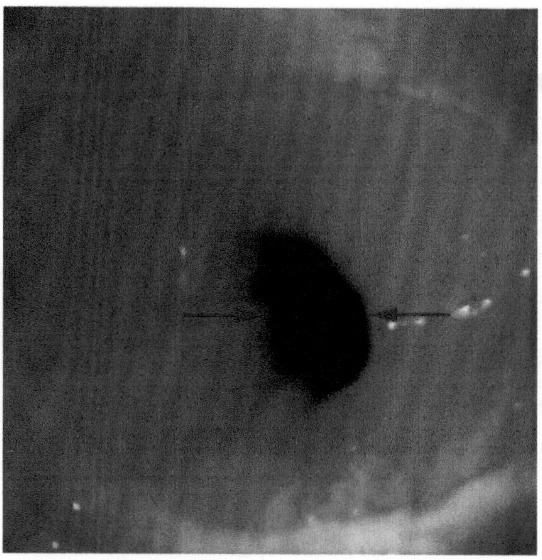

Fig. 3. The diaphragm forms a circumferential compression at the distal aspect of the esophagus.

POTENTIAL COMPLICATIONS AND THEIR MANAGEMENT

No major complications have been reported by otolarygologists performing TNE. Among the thousands of TNE cases that have been performed, 1 case of esophageal perforation has been reported by a gastroenterologist.[7] Fortunately, even minor complications are rare. Epistaxis rates are between 0.85% and 2% and vasovagal events have occurred in 0.3%.[6,25]

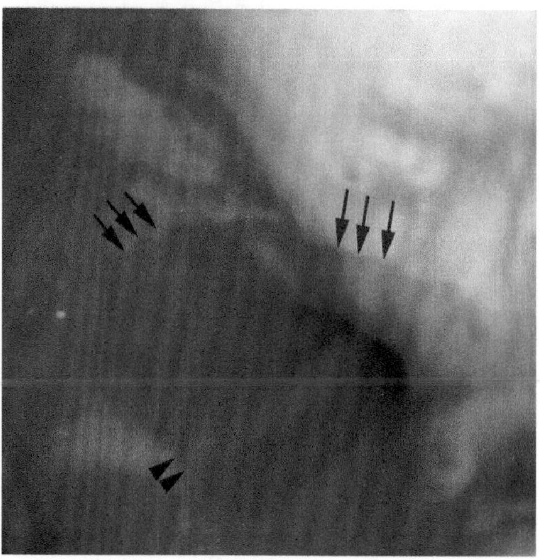

Fig. 4. At the squamocolumnar junction the squamous epithelium of the esophagus (*gray-white*) meets the gastric mucosa (*salmon pink*).

Table 2
A Brief Review of Current TNE Literature

Title	Pt Population	Pt #	Results
Role of flexible TNE and patient education in the management of globus pharyngeus[28]	Globus sensation/dysphagia	36	100% completed procedure 1 case of epistaxis Significant improvement in symptoms after TNE/treatment with a proton pump inhibitor
TNE findings: Interspecialty comparison[27]	Throat symptoms (ie, hoarseness, cough, dysphagia, globus)	50	100% completed procedure Otolaryngologist were more likely than an esophagologist to find an abnormality 86% agreement for Barrett's esophagus between otolaryngologist and esophagologist 50% of patients had normal examinations, Barrett's esophagus was noted in 12% and hiatal hernia in 32% of patients on review by esophagologist
Feasibility, safety, acceptability, and yield of office-based, screening TNE[26]	Participants recruited at random (40–85 years old) from general medicine clinic; patients with previously diagnosed pathology were excluded	426	422 (99%) completed examination No major adverse events 38% had esophageal findings that changed management (34% erosive esophagitis and 4% Barrett's esophagus)
TNE: White-light versus narrowband imaging[29]	LPR	111	13.5% with biopsy-proven Barrett's esophagus 2.7% with dysplasia on biopsy 12.1% and 15.1% rates of Barrett's esophagus detected with white light versus narrow band imaging, respectively
Unsedated TNE: A new technique for accurately detecting and grading esophageal varices in cirrhotic patients[13]	Patients with h/o cirrhosis (patients with h/o variceal bleeding excluded)	15	No significant difference in patient tolerance of TNE versus conventional Both modalities performed on all patients with 100% agreement rate for esophageal and gastric varices between blinded endoscopists 1 case of epistaxis

TNE – Revisited (>700 consecutive cases)[6]	Patients meeting TNE indication (LPR, dysphagia, screening, biopsy, FB)	711	17 procedures aborted secondary to tight nasal vault Significant findings in 50% (most frequent esophagitis, hiatal hernia, and Barrett's) One case of self-limited vasovagal reaction No epistaxis requiring packing
Unsedated transnasal EGD in daily practice: Results with 1100 consecutive patients[25]	Patients meeting indications for esophagoscopy	1100	93.9% of patients were able to tolerate the procedure 2% incidence of epistaxis 0.3% incidence of vasovagal reaction 91% preferred TNE to transoral unsedated esophagoscopy
Detection of metachronous esophageal squamous carcinoma in patients with head and neck cancer with use of TNE[23]	Patients with previously treated head and neck cancer	293	Metachronous esophageal cancer was detected in 5.1% The prevalence rate was higher in patients with hypopharyngeal cancer (15.9%)
Transnasal small-caliber EGD for preoperative evaluation of the high-risk morbidly obese patient[14]	Morbidly obese patients scheduled for bariatric surgery	25	100% tolerated procedure Significant pathology was found in 56% Biopsies were indicated for 12 patients and successful in all 12 (100%)

Abbreviations: EGD, esophagogastroduodenoscopy; LPR, laryngopharyngealreflux.

REHABILITATION AND RECOVERY

No rehabilitation or recovery process is necessary.

OUTCOMES

Patients routinely do well after TNE. It the hands of otolaryngologists, TNE can be equated to transnasal flexible laryngoscopy as a benign, in office procedure. Major complications are exceedingly rare, and self-limiting, minor complications occur in less than 3%. The procedure can be performed rapidly (on average 3–6 minutes) and the patient can be discharged home immediately after. As mentioned, the sensitivity and specificity of TNE are high (89% sensitive, 97% specific). Of interest, approximately 50% of patients meeting indication for the procedure will have significant findings affecting treatment.[6,13,26,27]

CLINICAL RESULTS IN THE LITERATURE

TNE is a safe and efficacious procedure (**Table 2**). The ability to perform TNE in awake patients significantly decreases the morbidity of the procedure in comparison to CE. The ease with which the procedure may be performed has begun to lower the threshold for esophageal screening. The role of TNE in patient management continues to be defined, and with user experience the applications of TNE will likely continue to expand.

SUPPLEMENTARY DATA

Supplementary data related to this article can be found online at http://dx.doi.org/10.1016/j.otc.2012.08.016.

REFERENCES

1. Herrmann IF, Recio SA. Functional pharyngoesophagoscopy: a new technique for diagnostics and analyzing deglutition. Oper Tech Otolaryngol Head Neck Surg 1997;8:163–7.
2. Aviv JE, Takoudes TG, Ma G, et al. Office-based esophagoscopy: a preliminary report. Otolaryngol Head Neck Surg 2001;125:170–5.
3. Dean R, Dua K, Massey B, et al. A comparative study of unsedated transnasal esophagogastroduodenoscopy and conventional EGD. Gastrointest Endosc 1996;44:422–4.
4. Jobe BA, Hunter JG, Chang EY, et al. Office-based unsedated small-caliber endoscopy is equivalent to conventional sedated endoscopy in screening and surveillance for Barrett's esophagus: a randomized and blinded comparison. Am J Gastroenterol 2006;101:2693–703.
5. Saeian K, Staff DM, Vasilopoulos S, et al. Unsedated transnasal endoscopy accurately detects Barrett's metaplasia and dysplasia. Gastrointest Endosc 2002;56:472–8.
6. Postma GN, Cohen JT, Belafsky PC, et al. Transnasal esophagoscopy: revisited (over 700 consecutive cases). Laryngoscope 2005;115:321–3.
7. Zaman A, Hahn M, Hapke R, et al. A randomized trial of peroral versus transnasal unsedated endoscopy using an ultrathin videoendoscope. Gastrointest Endosc 1999;49:279–84.
8. Garcia RT, Cello JP, Nguyen MH, et al. Unsedated ultrathin EGD is well accepted when compared with conventional sedated EGD: a multicenter randomized trial. Gastroenterology 2003;125:1606–12.

9. Mulcahy HE, Riches A, Kiely M, et al. A prospective controlled trial of an ultrathin versus a conventional endoscope in unsedated upper gastrointestinal endoscopy. Endoscopy 2001;33:311–6.
10. Waring JP, Baron TH, Hirota WK, et al, American Society for Gastrointestinal Endoscopy, Standards of Practice Committee. Guidelines for conscious sedation and monitoring during gastrointestinal endoscopy. Gastrointest Endosc 2003;58: 317–22.
11. Sharma VK, Nguyen CC, Crowell MD, et al. A national study of cardiopulmonary unplanned events after GI endoscopy. Gastrointest Endosc 2007;66:27–34.
12. Watts TL, Shahidzadeh R, Chaudhary A, et al. Cost saving of unsedated transnasal esophagosopy. Presented at the 87th Annual ABEA meeting. 2007. San Diego, April 26–27, 2007.
13. Saeian K, Staff D, Knox J, et al. Unsedated transnasal endoscopy: a new technique for accurately detecting and grading esophageal varices in cirrhotic patients. Am J Gastroenterol 2002;97(9):2246–9.
14. Alami RS, Schuster R, Friedland S, et al. Transnasal small-caliber esophagogastroduodenoscopy for preoperative evaluation of the high-risk morbidly obese patient. Surg Endosc 2007;21(5):758–60.
15. Rees CJ. In-office transnasal esophagoscope guided botulinum toxin injection of the lower esophageal sphincter. Curr Opin Otolaryngol Head Neck Surg 2007; 15(6):409–11.
16. Belafsky PC, Allen K, Castro-Del Rosario L, et al. Wireless pH testing as an adjunct to unsedated transnasal esophagoscopy: the safety and efficacy of transnasal telemetry capsule placement. Otolaryngol Head Neck Surg 2004; 131(1):26–8.
17. Pohl H, Welch HG. The role of overdiagnosis and reclassification in the marked increase of esophageal adenocarcinoma incidence. J Natl Cancer Inst 2005; 97(2):142–6.
18. Pohl H, Sirovich B, Welch HG. Esophageal adenocarcinoma incidence: are we reaching the peak? Cancer Epidemiol Biomarkers Prev 2010;19(6):1468–70.
19. Coppola D, Karl RC. Barrett's esophagus and Barrett's associated neoplasia: etiology and pathologic features. Cancer Control 1999;6(1):21–7.
20. Reavis KM, Morris CD, Gopal DV, et al. Laryngopharyngeal reflux symptoms better predict the presence of esophageal adenocarcinoma than typical gastroesophageal reflux symptoms. Ann Surg 2004;239:849–56.
21. Postma GN, Bach KK, Belafsky PC, et al. The role of transnasal esophagoscopy in head and neck oncology. Laryngoscope 2002;112(12):2242–3.
22. Farwell DG, Rees CJ, Mouadeb DA, et al. Esophageal pathology in patients after treatment for head and neck cancer. Otolaryngol Head Neck Surg 2010;143(3): 375–8.
23. Su YY, Fang FM, Chuang HC, et al. Detection of metachronous esophageal squamous carcinoma in patients with head and neck cancer with use of transnasal esophagoscopy. Head Neck 2010;32(6):780–5.
24. Postma GN, Belafsky PC, Aviv JE. Atlas of transnasal esophagoscopy. Philadelphia: Lippincott Williams & Wilkins; 2007.
25. Dumortier J, Napoleon B, Hedelius F, et al. Unsedated transnasal EGD in daily practice: results with 1100 consecutive patients. Gastrointest Endosc 2003; 57(2):198–204.
26. Peery AF, Hoppo T, Garman KS, et al, Barrett's Esophagus Risk Consortium. Feasibility, safety, acceptability, and yield of office-based, screening transnasal esophagoscopy (with video). Gastrointest Endosc 2012;75(5):945–53.e2.

27. Falcone MT, Garrett CG, Slaughter JC, et al. Transnasal esophagoscopy findings: interspecialty comparison. Otolaryngol Head Neck Surg 2009;140(6):812–5.
28. Cheng CC, Fang TJ, Lee TJ, et al. Role of flexible transnasal esophagoscopy and patient education in the management of globus pharyngeus. J Formos Med Assoc 2012;111(3):171–5.
29. O'Brien TJ, Parham K. Transnasal esophagoscopy: white-light versus narrow-band imaging. Ann Otol Rhinol Laryngol 2008;117(12):886–90.

Office-Based Botulinum Toxin Injections

Manish D. Shah, MD, MPhil[a], Michael M. Johns III, MD[b,*]

KEYWORDS

• Botulinum toxin • Botox • Spasmodic dysphonia • Dystonia • Ambulatory surgery

KEY POINTS

- Office-based botulinum toxin injections are well-tolerated and easy to perform with appropriate equipment and experience.
- Botulinum toxin injections have been demonstrated to be effective in the treatment of various laryngeal disorders, including spasmodic dysphonia (SD), vocal tremor, bilateral vocal fold paralysis, paradoxic vocal fold motion, ventricular dysphonia, and cricopharyngeal achalasia.

INTRODUCTION

Botulinum toxin is a natural neurotoxin produced by clostridial bacterial species that causes muscular paralysis.[1] The primary mechanism of action of the toxin is via inhibition of calcium-dependent exocytosis and release of acetylcholine at the neuromuscular junction. Other indirect mechanisms of action may also explain the clinical effect of the toxin. Inhibition of intramuscular gamma motor neurons and lack of feedback to motor neurons due to muscle weakening may have an effect on afferent feedback to the central nervous system.[1] The effect of botulinum toxin is reversible because the nerve terminals do recover the ability to release acetylcholine into the neuromuscular junction.

There are seven serotypes of the botulinum toxin; only type A and type B have been developed for clinical use in humans:

- Type A has the longest duration of effect and diffuses less from the point of injection compared with type B. These differences may be secondary to differences in the preparation of the toxin as opposed to inherent differences in the serotypes themselves.[1]

[a] Department of Otolaryngology Head & Neck Surgery, University of Toronto, Canada; [b] Department of Otolaryngology Head & Neck Surgery, Emory University, 550 Peachtree Street NE, Suite 9-4400, Atlanta, GA 30308, USA

* Corresponding author.

E-mail address: michael.johns2@emory.edu

Otolaryngol Clin N Am 46 (2013) 53–61

http://dx.doi.org/10.1016/j.otc.2012.08.017 oto.theclinics.com

- The dosing differs significantly between type A and type B preparations. The focus of information in this article is based on the use of type A (Botox, Allergan Irvine, USA; Dysport, Ipsen, Ltd, Slough, UK).

There are numerous indications for botulinum toxin injection in the treatment of laryngeal disorders. The most common use of botulinum toxin is for the treatment of spasmodic dysphonia (SD), a focal dystonia affecting the laryngeal musculature. SD is classified as primarily adductor (ADSD), abductor (ABSD), or of a mixed nature. Distinguishing between these conditions can often be subtle and difficult (a fully detailed discussion of this is beyond the scope of this article). This determination is essential to the effective treatment with targeted botulinum toxin injections, which is the mainstay of management for this condition.[2] The thyroarytenoid-lateral cricoarytenoid (TA-LCA) muscle complex is targeted for ADSD while the posterior cricoarytenoid (PCA) muscle is targeted for ABSD.

Essential tremor and age-related disease that involves involuntary muscle contraction can affect the upper aerodigestive tract muscles with varying degrees of impact on voice production. Symptoms can range from mild to severe vocal disability. Systemic pharmacologic intervention for vocal tremor is generally ineffective; however, botulinum toxin injections have proven to be helpful in selected patients.[3,4] Tremor can also be observed in other neurologic conditions, such as Parkinson's disease, and can coexist with SD.[5]

Plica ventricularis refers to hyperfunction of the supraglottic larynx and excessive adduction of the false vocal folds with phonation, resulting in poor voice quality. This may arise secondary to an underlying pathologic condition at the level of the true vocal folds that is resulting in glottal insufficiency or impaired vocal fold vibration. However, it may also be functional in origin.[6] Traditional management typically involves a combination of treatment of any underlying cause at the level of the true vocal folds and aggressive voice therapy. Voice therapy aims to teach patients to reduce false vocal fold phonation and resume phonation with the true vocal folds; however, some patients may continue to have problems despite aggressive therapy. In these cases, weakening the contraction of the false folds, that is, the aryepiglottic muscle, via a botulinum toxin injection may help facilitate more effective therapy.[5,6]

The use of botulinum toxin has been recently described as a potential treatment of patients with bilateral vocal fold paralysis and posterior glottic stenosis.[7] By weakening the TA-LCA muscle complex, the PCA muscle has less opposition and can lead to a more lateralized position of the vocal folds, thus improving the caliber of the airway. Although this technique had good success in treating patients with bilateral vocal fold paralysis, results in patients with PGS were mixed.[7]

The management of vocal fold granulomas can be challenging and typically involves voice therapy and aggressive management of laryngopharyngeal reflux. Surgery plays a minimal role because it is often ineffective.[8] Various investigators have found that botulinum toxin injection into the ipsilateral vocal fold can be an effective adjunctive treatment of recalcitrant granulomas[8–10] by preventing forceful contact between the arytenoids during phonation and coughing.

Paradoxic vocal fold motion is characterized by the inappropriate adduction of the true vocal folds during inspiration. There are a wide range of proposed causes and treatments[11,12] (further discussion is beyond the scope of this article). It is often a very difficult condition to treat effectively and botulinum toxin injections have been proposed as an effective adjunctive treatment in severe or refractory cases.[11,13,14]

Botulinum toxin injections into the cricopharyngeus muscle can also be effective in the treatment of dysphagia secondary to increased tone and delayed relaxation of this muscle.[15–17] This technique can also be used as a predictor for which patients will benefit from a surgical cricopharyngeal myotomy.[15]

Botulinum toxin injections are contraindicated in patients who are pregnant or breastfeeding, have concurrent neuromuscular diseases (eg, myasthenia gravis), are receiving concurrent aminoglycoside treatment, or have a known sensitivity to botulinum toxin or any of the compounds contained in the toxin preparation.

PREOPERATIVE PLANNING, PREPARATION, AND PATIENT POSITIONING

Botox is supplied as a vacuum-dried concentrated powder in 100-unit vials and it is reconstituted with sterile normal saline. The authors prefer to use 4.0 mL of saline for the reconstitution, which provides a dose of 2.5 U/0.1 mL. This can be further diluted based upon the dose required; the preferred injection volume is 0.1 to 0.2 mL per vocal fold.

Some investigators prefer not to use local anesthesia for percutaneous injections. The authors, however, have found that the use of a small amount of injected 1% lidocaine in the skin and subcutaneous tissue improves patient comfort. Topical anesthesia of the larynx is typically not required, unless the planned approach involves the electrode needle piercing the endolaryngeal mucosa (eg, for PCA muscle injections; see later discussion).

Percutaneous injections should be guided via electromyography to maximize the accuracy of injection location. Needle placement is crucial to achieve accurate distribution of the toxin. The EMG machine must be appropriately set-up and calibrated along with placement of ground and reference electrodes before starting any injection procedure and the physician must be comfortable with basic EMG interpretation to use this technique. EMG-guided injections should be done with a 26-gauge or 27-gauge needle electrode. Injections can be done without EMG guidance[18,19] by using laryngoscopic or visual guidance; however, the latter technique is less precise, in the opinion of the authors. EMG guidance allows for more precise injections, which should maximize the efficacy of the injected dose. Information here is focused on EMG-guided percutaneous techniques.

Counseling the patient regarding the nature of the procedure and expected time course of postinjection effects (see later discussion) is essential to maximize patient comfort and to minimize the risk of complications. The authors prefer patients to be in a comfortable seated position for all injections. The physician can be positioned on either side of the patient depending in the location of the injection and the physician's dominant hand.

PROCEDURAL APPROACH

TA-LCA Muscle Complex

The procedural approach is for the TA-LCA muscle complex is as follows.

- The needle is inserted 2 to 3 mm off of the midline through the cricothyroid membrane without piercing the endolaryngeal mucosa.
- The needle should be directed superiorly and laterally such that it remains submucosal (**Fig. 1**). The needle can be inserted into the airway first, then directed superiorly and laterally; however, this is uncomfortable for the patient and can elicit coughing.
- There will be a visible and audible insertion potential when the needle enters the muscle and asking the patient to phonate should result in brisk recruitment. The toxin should be injected at this point and the needle withdrawn.

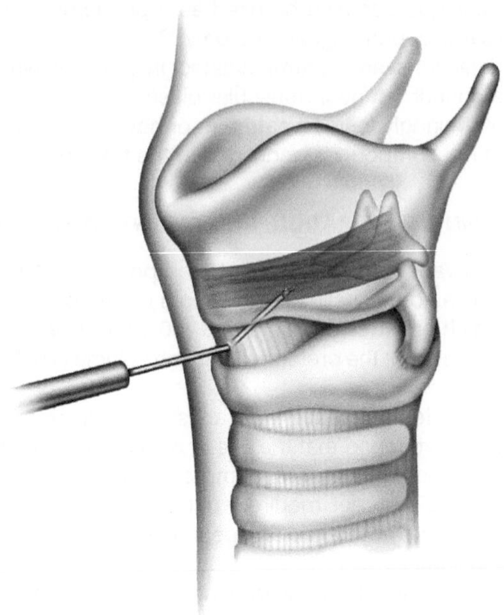

Fig. 1. Insertion of EMG needle through the cricothyroid membrane into the TA-LCA muscle complex. (*Reprinted from* Sulica L, Blitzer A. Botulinum toxin treatment of spasmodic dysphonia. Oper Techniques Otolaryngol 2004;15:76–80; with permission.)

There is no standard dose for treatment of ADSD; however, 0.625 to 2.5 units per vocal fold would be typical doses. Injections are typically done bilaterally; however, some investigators have found success with unilateral injections.[2,20] The dose should be reassessed and altered at each subsequent reinjection based on the voice benefits achieved and side-effects experienced with the previous injection. A reasonable starting dose for the first injection is 1.25 to 2.5 units. Vocal tremor is also typically treated with bilateral TA-LCA muscle complex injections, although a lower dose is typically used.[19]

The TA-LCA complex can also be injected for the treatment of vocal fold granulomas. The ipsilateral muscle complex is injected with the toxin; doses of 1.25 to 20 units have been described.[8–10] Finally, paradoxical vocal fold motion (PVFM),[11,13,14] bilateral vocal fold paralysis, or posterior glottic stenosis[7] can be treated with bilateral or unilateral TA-LCA injections.

PCA Muscle

There are two approaches for injection of the PCA muscle for ABSD: retrolaryngeal or translaryngeal.

Retrolaryngeal

- For the retrolaryngeal approach (**Fig. 2**), the larynx is gently rotated by the physician to expose the posterior aspect of the larynx on the side to be injected.
- The needle should be directed posterior to the posterior border of the thyroid cartilage, near its inferior extent, until it hits the cricoid cartilage.

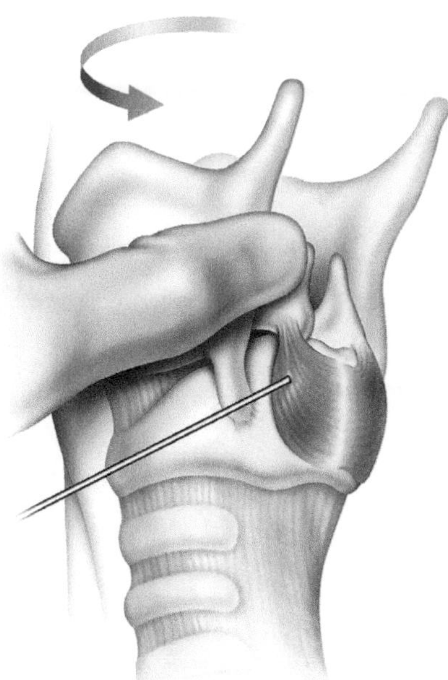

Fig. 2. Retrocricoid approach for PCA muscle injection. (*Reprinted from* Sulica L, Blitzer A. Botulinum toxin treatment of spasmodic dysphonia. Oper Techniques Otolaryngol 2004;15:76–80; with permission.)

- The needle should then be slightly withdrawn and the patient is asked to sniff; brisk recruitment confirms position and the toxin can be injected.

Translaryngeal

- The translaryngeal approach (**Fig. 3**) requires topical anesthesia of the laryngeal mucosa because the needle will pierce the endolaryngeal mucosa.
- The needle enters the larynx in the midline through the cricothyroid membrane and is directed toward the side to be injected.
- The needle then needs to be pushed through the posterior cricoid cartilage lamina.
- The PCA is immediately on the posterior surface of the cartilage (as with the retrolaryngeal approach); sniffing should elicit brisk recruitment and the injection can be made.
- Plugs of cartilage can block the needle and significant force may be required to expel these cartilage plugs. This approach may be impossible in older patients with significant calcification of the laryngeal cartilages.

For ABSD, typically, one PCA muscle is injected with 3.75 to 5 units and vocal fold mobility is evaluated 2 weeks later. The dose for the second vocal fold will be determined by the mobility of the previously injected vocal fold. An immobile fold will prompt a very small dose on the contralateral side, whereas a fold with near normal mobility allows for a higher contralateral injection.[2,19] Asymmetric dosing is advisable for ABSD because of the risk of airway compromise.

False Vocal Folds

Supraglottic Botox injections can be effective for a variety of conditions, including essential tremor and plica ventricularis. There are two approaches: peroral and via

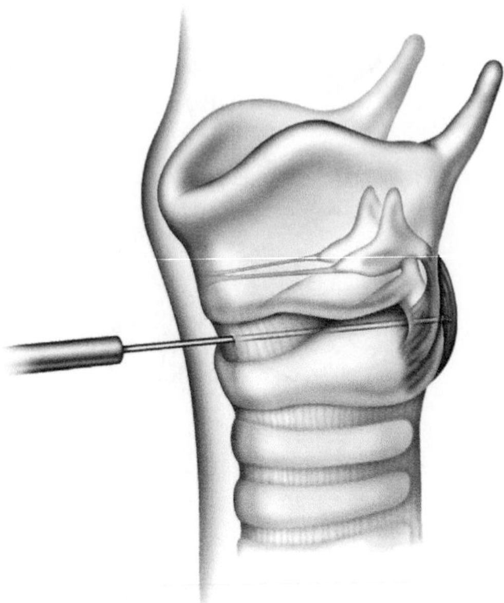

Fig. 3. Transcricoid approach for PCA muscle injection. (*Reprinted from* Sulica L, Blitzer A. Botulinum toxin treatment of spasmodic dysphonia. Oper Techniques Otolaryngol 2004;15:76–80; with permission.)

the working channel of a flexible laryngoscope. The latter approach is generally better tolerated by most patients, but requires a flexible scope with a working channel and a fine-gauge injection needle designed to be passed through this channel.

For the peroral approach, after appropriate laryngopharyngeal anesthesia, the patient's tongue is held by the patient or the surgeon and the larynx is visualized with either a flexible or rigid scope.

The rigid scope offers the advantage of eliminating the need for an assistant because the patient holds their own tongue while the surgeon holds the scope in one hand and the needle for injection in the other.

Use of the flexible scope held by an assistant, however, is generally better tolerated by the patient and allows the surgeon to have bimanual control of the needle.

A long curved needle is required. The curved orotracheal injection instrument (Medtronic Xomed, Jacksonville, FL, USA) is designed for peroral injections with 27-gauge needles. Other long needles designed for injection during direct laryngoscopy in the operating room can often be bent to the required shape for peroral injection (eg, 24 gauge rigid injection needle, Merz Aesthetics, Franksville, WI, USA). The needle is advanced to the injection site through the oral cavity and past the oropharyngeal structures. Needle placement can be easily controlled and visualized, allowing for a precise injection of the false vocal folds. Typically, 5 to 7.5 units of Botox are injected into each fold.[5,19]

This technique can also be used to inject the TA-LCA muscle complex if EMG guidance is not available. Furthermore, it can be used to inject the interarytenoid muscle, which has been described in the management of ADSD and vocal tremor.[21]

Cricopharyngeus

The cricopharyngeus muscle can be injected percutaneously using EMG guidance. The muscle is lateral and posterior to the cricoid cartilage. The needle is inserted until it hits the cricoid cartilage and is then incrementally advanced posteriorly using the needle to palpate the cartilage. Once the needle is posterior to the cartilage, the muscle is located by identification of basal resting action potentials that cease with swallowing and do not change with sniffing (to avoid inadvertent PCA injection). Typically, only unilateral injections are done to avoid potential for bilateral PCA paralysis and resultant airway compromise.

IMMEDIATE POSTPROCEDURAL CARE

Patients can be discharged from clinic immediately following the injections. They should be educated regarding the expected outcomes as outlined following.

POTENTIAL COMPLICATIONS WITH OFFICE-BASED LARYNGEAL BOTULINUM TOXIN INJECTIONS

Office-based botulinum toxin injections are generally well-tolerated and safe.

Patient Discomfort or Vasovagal Episode

Very rarely, the procedure may have to be terminated due to patient discomfort or a vasovagal episode. The needle insertion itself can potentially cause severe coughing or laryngospasm and can result in vocal fold hemorrhage.

Inappropriate Injection Causing Muscle Weakening

Inappropriate injection, either the wrong location or an excessive dose, can result in adverse effects. Excessive weakening of the intended muscle or unintended weakening of adjacent muscles can be very problematic, stressing the importance of appropriate dosing and location of delivery. Excessive weakening of the TA-LCA muscle complex can result in a higher risk of significant aspiration, whereas excessive bilateral PCA muscle weakening can result in stridor and potential airway compromise. Excessive bilateral PCA weakness has even been described with TA-LCA injections, presumably from diffusion of the injected toxin.[22]

Systemic Effects

Systemic effects from botulinum toxin have been described,[1,23] but such effects would be highly unlikely at the typical doses used to treat laryngeal disorders.

REHABILITATION AND RECOVERY

Botulinum toxin injections result in maximal muscle weakness for 1 to 2 weeks followed by milder weakness for 2 to 4 months, depending on the dose and accuracy of injection. Patients should be counseled appropriately about the timeline of these effects. Those who undergo TA-LCA injections should expect to experience some vocal breathiness and can have mild symptoms of aspiration, especially with thin liquids, during the period of maximal weakness. Patients who undergo a bilateral staged PCA injection for ABSD should be warned about the potential for dyspnea and stridor following the second injection. As the effect of the toxin diminishes, patients' symptoms will return and repeat injections will be required.

OUTCOMES AND CLINICAL RESULTS IN THE LITERATURE

Botulinum toxin injections are widely accepted as the primary treatment modality for spasmodic dysphonia.[5] There are many subtle variations to clinical practice in terms of dose and schedule (detailed discussion is beyond the scope of this article).

Although the cycle of muscle recovery and repeat injection does result in fluctuation in voice quality and side-effects, the results are generally very favorable.[5,24–26] Vocal tremor is more difficult to treat with botulinum toxin injections because it can affect many of the muscles of the upper aerodigestive tract. However, studies have found that bilateral TA-LCA injections can help improve voice quality.[3–5] Mixed efficacy has been found in treating PVFM,[11,13,14] vocal fold granulomas,[8–10] plica ventricularis,[5,6] bilateral vocal fold paralysis,[7] and cricopharyngeal dysphagia.[15–17]

SUMMARY

Botulinum toxin injections are effective treatment of numerous laryngeal disorders. Adequate physician training and appropriate patient selection and preparation are essential to ensuring safe and successful injections.

REFERENCES

1. Aoki KR. Pharmacology of botulinum neurotoxins. Oper Techniques Otolaryngol Head Neck Surg 2004;15:81–5.
2. Sulica L, Blitzer A. Botulinum toxin treatment of spasmodic dysphonia. Oper Techniques Otolaryngol Head Neck Surg 2004;15:76–80.
3. Adler CH, Bansberg SF, Hentz JG, et al. Botulinum toxin type A for treating voice tremor. Arch Neurol 2004;61:1416–20.
4. Warrick P, Dromey C, Irish J, et al. The treatment of essential voice tremor with botulinum toxin A: a longitudinal case report. J Voice 2000;14:410–21.
5. Zalvan C, Blitzer A. Using botulinum therapy in the laryngopharynx. Oper Techniques Otolaryngol 2004;15:86–9.
6. Maryn Y, De Bodt MS, Van Cauwenberge P. Ventricular dysphonia: clinical aspects and therapeutic options. Laryngoscope 2003;113:859–66.
7. Ekbom DC, Garrett CG, Yung KC, et al. Botulinum toxin injections for new onset bilateral vocal fold motion impairment in adults. Laryngoscope 2010;12:758–63.
8. Zeitels SM, Casiano RR, Gardner GM, et al. Management of common voice problems: committee report. Otolaryngol Head Neck Surg 2002;126:333–48.
9. Orloff LA, Goldman SN. Vocal fold granuloma: successful treatment with botulinum toxin. Otolaryngol Head Neck Surg 1999;121:410–3.
10. Nasri S, Sercarz JA, McAlpin T, et al. Treatment of vocal fold granuloma using botulinum toxin type A. Laryngoscope 1995;105:585–8.
11. Altman KW, Mirza N, Ruiz C, et al. Paradoxical vocal fold motion: presentation and treatment options. J Voice 2000;14:99–103.
12. Maschka DA, Bauman NM, McCray PB Jr, et al. A classification scheme for paradoxical vocal cord motion. Laryngoscope 1997;107(11 Pt 1):1429–35.
13. Chalhoub M, Harris K, Sasso L, et al. The use of botox in the treatment of post cardiac surgery paradoxical vocal cord movement. Heart Lung Circ 2011;20: 602–4.
14. Maillard I, Schweizer V, Broccard A, et al. Use of botulinum toxin type A to avoid tracheal intubation or tracheostomy in severe paradoxical vocal cord movement. Chest 2000;118:874–7.
15. Ahsan SF, Meleca RJ, Dworkin JP. Botulinum toxin injection of the cricopharyngeus muscle for the treatment of dysphagia. Otolaryngol Head Neck Surg 2000; 122:691–5.
16. Blitzer A, Brin MF. Use of botulinum toxin for diagnosis and management of cricopharyngeal achalasia. Otolaryngol Head Neck Surg 1997;116:328–30.

17. Chiu MJ, Chang YC, Hsiao TY. Prolonged effect of botulinum toxin injection in the treatment of cricopharyngeal dysphagia: case report and literature review. Dysphagia 2004;19:52–7.
18. Green DC, Berke GS, Ward PH, et al. Point-touch technique of botulinum toxin injection for the treatment of spasmodic dysphonia. Ann Otol Rhinol Laryngol 1992;101:883–7.
19. Sulica L. Botulinum toxin injection of the larynx. In: Rosen CA, Simpson CB, editors. Operative techniques in laryngology. Berlin: Springer; 2008. p. 221–7.
20. Bielamowicz S, Stager SV, Badillo A, et al. Unilateral versus bilateral injections of botulinum toxin in patients with adductor spasmodic dysphonia. J Voice 2002;16: 117–23.
21. Kendall KA, Leonard RJ. Interarytenoid muscle botox injection for treatment of adductor spasmodic dysphonia with vocal tremor. J Voice 2011;25:114–9.
22. Venkatesan NN, Johns MM, Hapner ER, et al. Abductor paralysis after botox injection for adductor spasmodic dysphonia. Laryngoscope 2010;120:1177–80.
23. Crowner BE, Torres-Russotto D, Carter AR, et al. Systemic weakness after therapeutic injections of botulinum toxin a: a case series and review of the literature. Clin Neuropharmacol 2010;33:243–7.
24. Braden MN, Johns MM 3rd, Klein AM, et al. Assessing the effectiveness of botulinum toxin injections for adductor spasmodic dysphonia: clinician and patient perception. J Voice 2010;24:242–9.
25. Novakovic D, Waters HH, D'Elia JB, et al. Botulinum toxin treatment of adductor spasmodic dysphonia: longitudinal functional outcomes. Laryngoscope 2011; 121:606–12.
26. Rubin AD, Wodchis WP, Spak C, et al. Longitudinal effects of Botox injections on voice-related quality of life (V-RQOL) for patients with adductory spasmodic dysphonia: part II. Arch Otolaryngol Head Neck Surg 2004;130:415–20.

Office Airway Surgery

Peter C. Belafsky, MD, MPH, PhD*, Maggie A. Kuhn, MD

KEYWORDS

• Airway • Bronchoscopy • Tracheoscopy • Surgical procedures • Awake surgery

KEY POINTS

- Numerous diagnostic and therapeutic airway procedures may be performed on awake patients in the otolaryngologist's office.
- With careful patient selection and pre-procedural counseling, acceptance and tolerance of unsedated airway procedures are high.
- Published outcomes demonstrate efficacy and safety comparable to their sedated or operating room counterparts and are accompanied by lower costs and more expeditious patient recovery.

OVERVIEW

Airway compromise results from numerous causes presenting with a relatively limited symptom profile, including dyspnea, stridor, hoarseness, and hemoptysis. Pathology of the upper airway can be categorized as

- Idiopathic
- Inflammatory (granulomatous diseases, polychondritis)
- Neoplastic (benign, malignant, metastatic)
- Acquired stenosis or vocal fold paralysis (trauma, postintubation, tracheotomy, postsurgical)
- Congenital

The use of mechanical ventilator support, endotracheal intubation, and tracheotomy expanded significantly during the mid-twentieth century amidst the polio epidemic and continues to be a major constituent in the care of hospitalized patients who are surviving complex injuries and disease. Subglottic and tracheal stenosis resulting from these measures account for a large percentage of patients with symptomatic airway obstruction. Rates of postintubation subglottic stenosis are estimated at

Department of Otolaryngology/Head and Neck Surgery, Center for Voice and Swallowing, School of Medicine, University of California at Davis, 2521 Stockton Boulevard, Suite 7200, Sacramento, CA 95817, USA
* Corresponding author.
E-mail address: pbelafsky@sbcglobal.net

Otolaryngol Clin N Am 46 (2013) 63–74
http://dx.doi.org/10.1016/j.otc.2012.08.018
oto.theclinics.com
0030-6665/13/$ – see front matter

0.9% to 8.3%.[1,2] Recognized factors increasing a ventilated patient's risk of airway stenosis include duration of intubation and size of endotracheal tube.[3]

Airway narrowing may exist for a generous period of time before the obstruction becomes apparent, and this is particularly true in less-active patients who lead sedentary lives. Typically, narrowing of the airway must reach 30% before symptoms appear at rest.[4] The workup of such patients might include imaging and pulmonary function testing, but of paramount importance is endoscopic assessment, necessary for locating, characterizing, and often treating airway obstruction. Treatment options for laryngotracheal stenosis include observation, endoscopic dilation with or without laser assistance, stent placement, open airway surgery, and tracheotomy.[5]

INDICATIONS

The primary indication for office-based airway surgery is the treatment of stenosis, the most common cause being idiopathic subglottic stenosis. Acquired tracheal or more distal stenosis and glottic webs are the second and third most common indications for in-office airway procedures. **Fig. 1** displays the most common reasons that bring patients to our center for office-based airway surgery.

Other indications for office-based airway intervention include biopsy of suspicious lesions, secondary tracheoesophageal puncture, foreign body retrieval,[6] and treatment of recurrent respiratory papillomatosis. Furthermore, office-based airway procedures are ideal for those in whom sedated or operative procedures are difficult or impossible because of significant comorbidity, cervical spine disease, morbid obesity, maxillofacial challenges, or extensive laryngotracheal papillomas.

PREOPERATIVE PLANNING

Before office-based airway surgery, patients should be counseled and prepared on what to expect. If undue anxiety is encountered, the procedure should be performed under intravenous sedation or general anesthesia. It is helpful to reassure patients that "they are in control" and that they may terminate the procedure at any time should they experience significant discomfort. Maintaining communication with the patient during the procedure, placing a hand on the patient's shoulder, and making intermittent eye

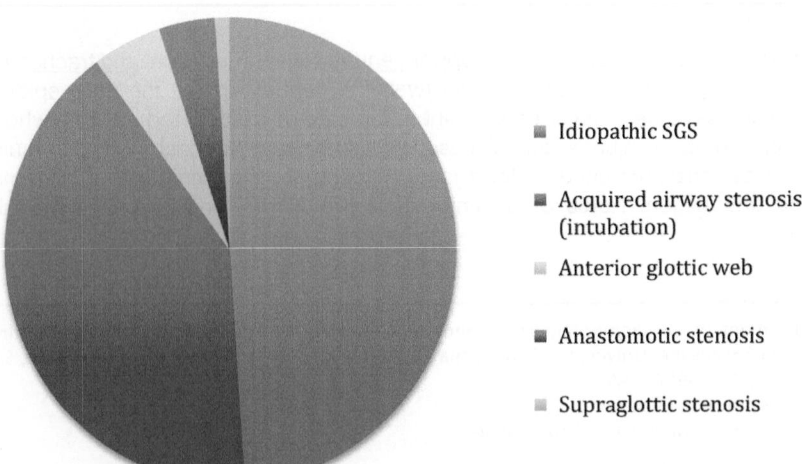

Fig. 1. Indications for office-based airway surgery. SGS, subglottic stenosis.

contact when possible helps ensure patient comfort and a successful outcome. A nurse opposite the endoscopist holding the patient's hand or explaining the steps of the procedure into the patient's ear is also beneficial in maximizing patient comfort and reducing anxiety.

Office-based tracheobronchoscopy, laser airway surgery, and balloon tracheoplasty may induce hemodynamic changes and exacerbate reactive airway disease. Mean arterial pressure, heart rate, cardiac index, and pulmonary arteriolar occlusion pressure have all been shown to significantly increase during bronchoscopy.[7] Surgery on the glottis and trachea can stimulate a reflex sympathetic discharge and result in ST segment alterations as well as significant decreases in forced expiratory volume in one second, forced vital capacity, and peak inspiratory and expiratory flow.[7–9] Caution must be exercised when considering office-based airway surgery on patients with cardiopulmonary disease, and the possibility of hemodynamic changes associated with awake procedures must be weighed against the risks of intravenous sedation or general anesthesia.

PREPARATION AND PATIENT POSITIONING

In addition to patient counseling and informed consent, adequate preparation for an office-based airway procedure requires assembling appropriate equipment and staff as well as achieving sufficient topical anesthesia. Any of a variety of endoscopes may be selected for the procedure; preferred are ultrathin distal chip bronchoscopes or esophagoscopes. The patient is comfortably seated upright in a standard examination chair positioned in front of a viewing screen linked to a recording system. When an intervention is anticipated, appropriate equipment, such as biopsy forceps, brushes, guide wires, laser fibers, and hydrostatic balloons, should be available. For patient safety and comfort, at least one, and ideally two assistants are required for office-based airway surgery.

Our technique of patient preparation is aimed at maximizing comfort which is essential for a successful procedure.

- First, topical anesthesia of 6 mL of 4% lidocaine is delivered via nebulizer, which is well tolerated and takes approximately 10 minutes to dispense (**Fig. 2**).
- Then, the patient's more patent nasal cavity is topically anesthetized and decongested with a combination of 1:1 oxymetazoline hydrochloride (0.05%) and lidocaine hydrochloride topical solution (4%).
- Patients are instructed on what to expect throughout the duration of the procedure and informed that should they experience any undue discomfort to raise their hand to suspend the procedure.
- The ultrathin endoscope with a 2-mm working channel (Pentax VE-1530 transnasal esophagoscope, Pentax Precision Medical Co, KayPentax, Lincoln Park, NJ) is placed and positioned above the glottis.
- The endoscope is repeatedly lubricated with 2% viscous lidocaine throughout the procedure to maximize nasal comfort.
- An additional 2 mL of 2% lidocaine is sprayed via the working channel into the trachea, and 1 mL is sprayed onto the vocal folds while the patient performs a "laryngeal gargle" by producing a sustained vowel during administration of the anesthetic. This, in our experience, provides patients with adequate anesthesia for the procedure.

Other anesthetic techniques have been described for office-based airway procedures, including topical application through Abraham cannulas, transnasal red rubber

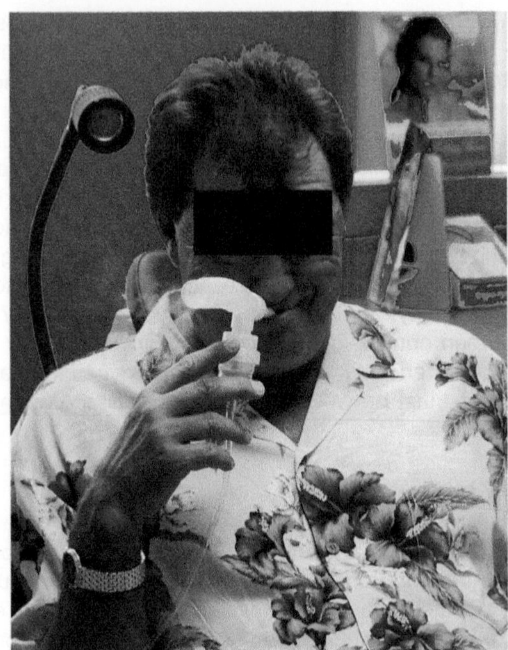

Fig. 2. Administration of 6 mL of 4% lidocaine via nebulizer before the procedure.

catheters,[10] or transcervical puncture,[11] as well as bilateral superior laryngeal nerve blocks, which are reserved for anticipated long dilation times.[12] Excessive anesthesia may lead to coughing caused by aspiration of saliva[13] and total administration of lidocaine must not exceed the patient's maximum allowable dose of 5 mg/kg.

PROCEDURAL APPROACH

Tracheoscopy and Bronchoscopy

The simplest and least invasive of in-office airway procedures are diagnostic evaluations of the upper airways. They require no additional equipment or personnel beyond an endoscope and the endoscopist.

- Tracheoscopy may be performed without additional topical anesthesia beyond what is used for traditional flexible laryngoscopy, whereby the endoscope is passed through abducted vocal folds during quick nasal inhalation for 2 seconds while the image is captured on video, which can be played at a later time.[14]
- Coughing is expected during the procedure, and the patient should be counseled of this beforehand.
- Additional anesthesia as described above affords a more extensive examination of the airways beyond the carina.
- Proximal third-order bronchi may be reached with a traditional flexible laryngoscope passed transorally.[10]

Balloon Tracheoplasty

- For treating tracheal stenosis, the patient is anesthetized as previously described, and the endoscope is passed through the more patent naris to the larynx then advanced gently into the trachea.

- After localization of the area in need of dilation, a flexible guide wire (Hydra Jagwire Guidewire, Boston Scientific, Natick, MA) is passed through the working channel of the endoscope and advanced past the area of stenosis (**Fig. 3**).
- The endoscope is then removed by withdrawing it while the first assistant gently advances the wire. This step requires an experienced endoscopist and assistant to avoid passing the guide wire too far into the distal airway, which would put the patient at risk for pneumothorax.
- Once the endoscope is removed, the guide wire is clamped with a hemostat by the assistant to stabilize its position and avoid migration.
- The endoscope is then immediately replaced through the same nasal cavity "sidecar" to the guide wire which is repositioned to 2 cm above the carina.
- With visualization of the tip of the guide wire, the balloon is advanced over the wire. The guide wire will need to be slowly withdrawn under endoscopic visualization to keep it from migrating into the distal airway as the balloon is advanced.
- Once the center of the balloon is positioned at the midpoint of the stenosis, the patient is informed that the dilation is about to take place (**Fig. 4**). The patient is asked to take a deep breath, exhale, and then hold his/her breath, effectively preventing an attempt to exhale against a completely obstructed airway. As discussed before the procedure, the patient is instructed to immediately raise a hand to signal discomfort or a desire to deflate the balloon and take a breath.
- The balloon is then inflated with isotonic sodium chloride solution to the desired diameter and kept inflated for 30 seconds or until the patient requests to stop (**Fig. 5**). Counting down from 30 by 5-second intervals while the balloon is inflated improves patient expectations, anxiety, and comfort.
- When the balloon is deflated, it is advanced into the distal trachea past the stenosis so that the patient can breathe. A deflated balloon left at the level of the stenosis or withdrawn proximally toward the larynx will limit the amount of available airway for the return of inspiration.
- If any blood is seen on the dilator, the procedure is terminated.
- After dilation, careful inspection of the dilated area is performed to assess for transmural injury.
- We routinely inject 0.2 to 0.6 mL of 40 mg/mL triamcinolone acetonide injectable suspension (**Fig. 6**) through a 4-mm sclerotherapy needle (Boston Scientific) after dilation.

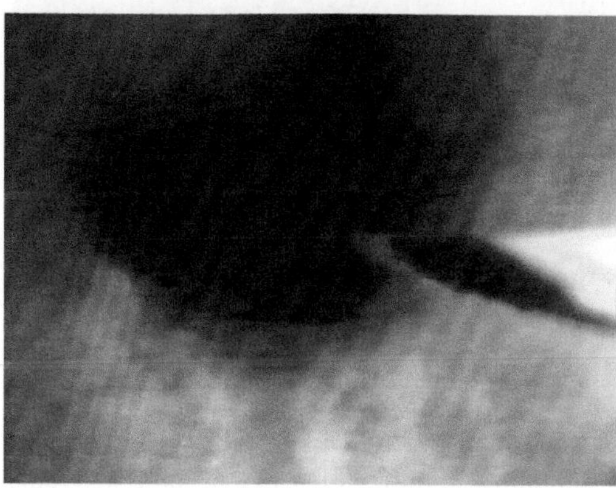

Fig. 3. Placement of the guide wire past the level of stenosis.

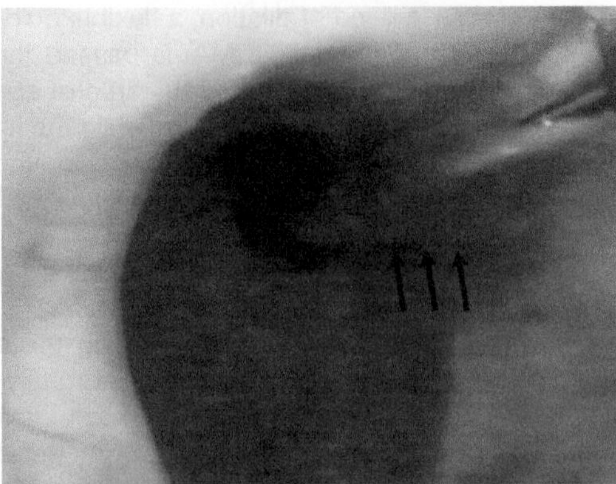

Fig. 4. Positioning the center of the balloon dilator at the midpoint of the stenosis.

Selection of balloon

We use controlled radial expansion (CRE) esophageal dilation balloons (Boston Scientific) for tracheal dilation. These balloons are 5 cm in length, and although shorter, 3 cm tracheal CRE dilators are available, we feel that the added length of the esophageal dilators is beneficial.

- The diameter of the stenosis is estimated by comparison with the known diameter of the endoscope tip (5.3 mm). Typically, the appropriate choice of balloon has a diameter that is 3 to 5 mm greater than that of the stenosis.
- Balloons may be inflated to three different diameters (eg, 8, 9, and 10 mm) with required pressures ranging from 3 to 8 atm depending on the desired balloon size.
- Because the balloons are transparent, the stricture may be visualized during the dilation.
- After the dilation is performed, the area of stenosis is inspected, and the decision is made to dilate to a larger diameter or to terminate the procedure.
- If further dilation is desired beyond the largest diameter of the balloon in use, it can be removed over the guide wire and a larger balloon can be positioned at the site.

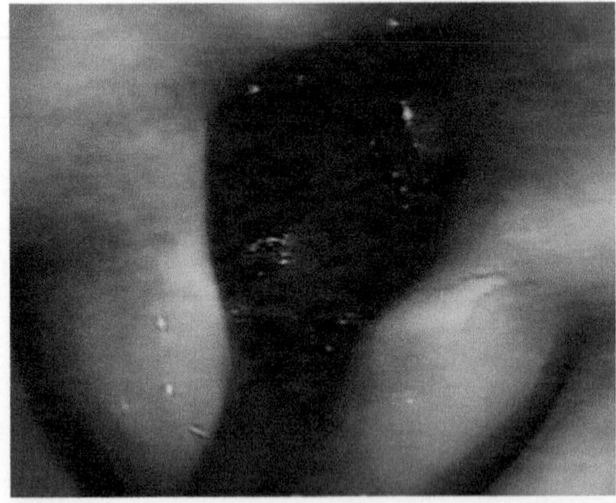

Fig. 5. Dilation of the subglottic stenosis with a 15 mm controlled radial expansion balloon dilator.

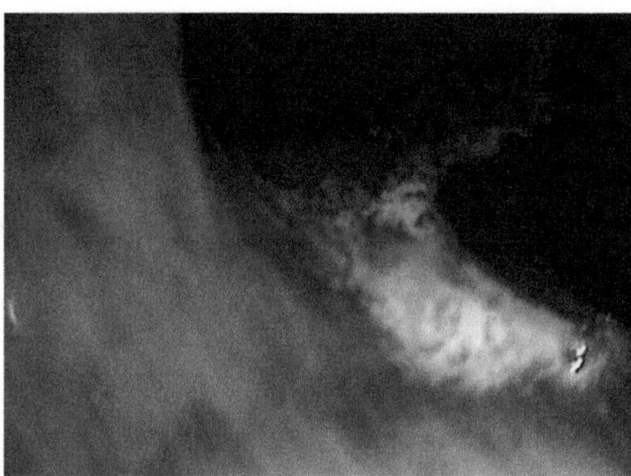

Fig. 6. Injection of triamcinolone into the area of stenosis after balloon tracheoplasty.

- The ultimate goal for tracheal dilation in adults is expansion to a diameter of 15 to 18 mm (45–54 Fr) depending on patient size and the diameter of the airway distal to the stenosis.

Laser Laryngoscopy and Tracheoplasty

Lasers may be used during office treatment of a variety of conditions including glottic webs, laryngotracheal papillomas and airway stenosis. The patient's airway and nasal cavity are anesthetized using the aforementioned technique. Multiple lasers are suitable for an office setting including CO2, Nd: YAG and pulse dye laser (PLD). We prefer the potassium titanyl phosphate laser (Aura XP KTP, American Medical Systems, Minnetonka, MN) in a contact mode. Laser parameters are selected depending on the desired tissue interaction. The laser fiber is advanced past the tip of the endoscope as contact between the endoscope and the laser fiber tip may damage the endoscope.

- For an anterior glottic web, the laser tip is positioned at the posterior aspect of the web, and with gentle anterior deflection on the endoscope, the laser fiber is moved from distal to proximal in a sweeping fashion along the web to reestablish the anterior commissure (**Figs. 7** and **8**). Multiple sweeps are performed until the tip of the fiber abuts the inner perichondrium of the thyroid cartilage at the anterior commissure.
- The laser may also be used to perform radial incisions in a mature subglottic or tracheal stenosis that is not amenable to balloon tracheoplasty alone. To accomplish this, the laser fiber is directed to make 4 quadrant radial incisions in a similar distal-to-proximal sweeping fashion.
- Balloon dilation is then performed.
- Steroids are routinely injected after the laser incision to promote postoperative healing.

POTENTIAL COMPLICATIONS AND THEIR MANAGEMENT

With proper patient selection and thoughtful execution of procedures, complications of airway surgery in the office are rare.

Vasovagal Reaction and Bronchospasm

The most common adverse events include vasovagal reaction and bronchospasm. In a review of office-based laser procedures of the larynx, only one patient of more than

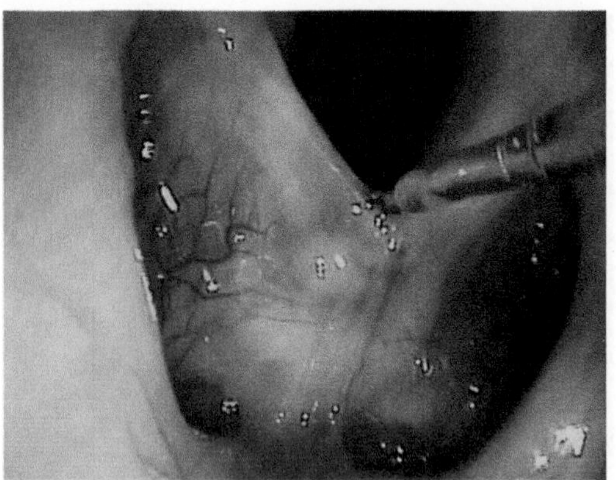

Fig. 7. Positioning of the laser fiber just before laser lysis of an anterior glottic web.

150 undergoing pulse dye laser (PDL) treatment experienced a vasovagal episode.[13] Bronchospasm occurs infrequently if the unsedated patient is adequately anesthetized and is more likely to occur during interventions of the distal airway. Lee and colleagues[15] reported the incidence of bronchospasm as less than 1% during bronchoscopic airway dilation. Manifestations include coughing, dyspnea or desaturation if pulse oximetry is monitored. Episodes are generally self-limited but may require temporary supplemental oxygen or a nebulized bronchodilator.

Equipment Failure

Equipment failures are rare as routine and frequent evaluation of instrumentation minimizes these occurrences. One such reported complication involved the PDL fiber tip breaking into the trachea during office treatment of subglottic granuloma.[13] It was successfully retrieved during the procedure with a cup forceps, and the patient had a normal recovery.

Superficial Tears

Superficial tears are frequent following tracheobronchial dilation. In one series of 124 procedures performed on 97 patients, 64 (51.6%) lacerations occurred. Of these,

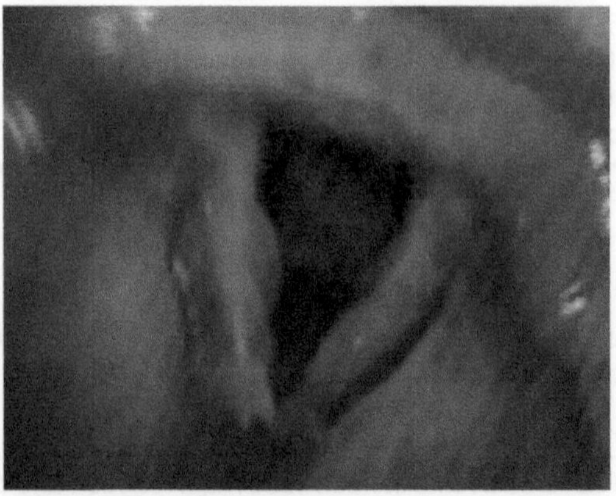

Fig. 8. Flexible endoscopic view 3 weeks after lysis of an anterior glottic web.

60 (94%) were superficial and 4 were deep.[16] The authors identified risk factors as female gender and stenosis resulting from tuberculosis or endotracheal/tracheotomy tube; they also found that patients who developed tears during the procedures experience longer periods of patency and less recurrence of stenosis than patients without laceration. In contrast, Lee and colleagues[15] found that although 15 patients with superficial tears following balloon dilation of benign stenoses experienced spontaneous resolution, more than half developed restenosis, granulation, or a cyst at the site of injury.

Airway Rupture and Deep Tracheal Lacerations

Airway dilation procedures, whether performed in an office setting or elsewhere, carry a risk of airway rupture. Complete or transmural disruption of the tracheobronchial tree is an exceptionally rare but potentially devastating complication of dilation for airway stenosis. As described in one report, dehiscence of the membranous trachea following dilation for a postintubation tracheal stenosis required repair with a bovine pericardial patch via thoracotomy.[17] Likewise, deep tracheal lacerations, which are not completely transmural, are uncommon and also less worrisome. Kim and colleagues[18] described two such injuries occurring during dilation of benign tracheal stenosis. Immediately after the procedure, patients complained of chest discomfort and hemoptysis; both were treated with oral antibiotics and healed spontaneously.

REHABILITATION AND RECOVERY

In-office airway procedures are performed without systemic sedatives, thereby obviating the need for continuous monitoring or an observed recovery period. Postprocedural care includes taking nothing by mouth for two hours to minimize the risk of aspiration while the effects of topical anesthesia subside. Patients are advised to immediately report symptoms of intractable cough, dyspnea, hemoptysis, and chest pain. Mild discomfort is common following airway interventions and is managed with non-narcotic pain medication. Patients are continued on pre-procedural reflux medications and precautions or such measures are initiated if not already in place.

OUTCOMES OF AMBULATORY AIRWAY SURGERY

Because of its recent description and cautious adoption by the otolaryngology community, reported outcomes for significant numbers of unsedated, in-office airway procedures are limited. Published outcomes of awake, endoscopic airway surgery are shown in **Table 1**.

Overall, patient tolerance of such procedures is high.[19] Of 30 patients undergoing unsedated transnasal tracheoscopy or bronchoscopy in an otolaryngology resident clinic, 29 were able to complete the procedure, and reported an average discomfort score of 3.4 (scale 1 to 10, range 1–8), with only 6 patients noting that they would have liked sedation during the procedure.[10] Likewise, in a retrospective review of more than 130 patients with upper aerodigestive pathologies undergoing endoscopy and PDL intervention, subjects reported an average overall comfort score of 7.4 (scale 1–10, SD 2.49).[20] Most of these patients who had previously undergone a fully sedated procedure in the operating room reported they would prefer that a repeat procedure be performed in-office.

As with other office-based laryngology procedures, in-office airway procedures seem to offer comparable efficacy for appropriately selected patients.[21] Series of patients undergoing awake, in-office PDL treatments for a variety of upper aerodigestive pathologies demonstrate high patient tolerance,[20] good efficacy,[22] and limited complications. Two recent reports underscore the feasibility of flexible, transnasal

Table 1
Clinical results in the literature

Report	Cases	Intervention	Outcomes Measured	Results	Complications
Leventhal et al,[24] 2009	16 patients with subglottic stenosis (66 procedures) sedated in OR	Flexible bronchoscopy & laser (Nd-YAG) tracheoplasty	1. Symptoms 2. Decannulation	1. Symptom reduction in 16 of 16 patients 2. Decannulation in 5 of 8 patients	Bleeding (n = 1)
Andrews et al,[23] 2007	18 patients with laryngotracheal stenosis (36 procedures) sedated in OR	Flexible bronchoscopy & laser (Nd-YAG)-assisted balloon tracheoplasty	None identified		None
Morris et al,[10] 2007	30 patients requiring diagnostic bronchoscopy (29 procedures) unsedated	Tracheobronchoscopy	1. Patient tolerance (discomfort scale 1–10) 2. Need for additional endoscopy	1. Average discomfort score of 3.4 2. 0 of 29	None
Rees et al,[20] 2006	131 patients with upper aerodigestive pathology (328 procedures) unsedated	Flexible endoscopy & laser (PDL) intervention	1. Patient tolerance (comfort scale 1–10)	1. Average comfort score of 7.4	Not reported
Postma et al,[22] 2004	10 patients with laryngeal granulomas unsedated	Flexible laryngoscopy & laser (PDL) excision	1. Lesion resolution	1. Complete resolution in 5 and partial resolution in 3 of 10	None
Hogikyan,[19] 1999	27 patients requiring diagnostic tracheoscopy (37 procedures) unsedated	Flexible tracheoscopy	1. Need for additional diagnostic test	1. None	None

Abbreviations: OR, operating room; PDL, pulse dye laser.

laser (Nd-YAG) bronchoscopies to treat stenosis in spontaneously breathing individuals.[23,24] Leventhal and colleagues[24] reported on patients with symptomatic or tracheotomy-dependent subglottic stenosis given light sedation to have procedures performed in the operating room. Although all patients required multiple procedures, each experienced a subjective improvement in reported symptoms, and 5 of 8 patients were able to have their tracheostomy tube or Montgomery stent removed. They reported a single complication of bleeding during one procedure that was ultimately controlled with electrocautery after the patient was intubated.

Initial studies examining costs related to office-based treatment of laryngeal papillomas demonstrate an overall cost savings of approximately $5000 per procedure.[25] Such savings may be extrapolated to in-office airway procedures that rely on similar anesthetic, endoscopic, and laser-based techniques. However, a recent review has uncovered poorer reimbursements for office-based procedures some less than 10% of their hospital-based counterparts.[26]

SUMMARY

Airway surgery can be performed safely and comfortably in the office without the need for intravenous sedation or general anesthesia. This affords patients numerous advantages, including enhanced safety, acceptable comfort, and shorter recovery with less time off from daily responsibilities. Furthermore, in-office, flexible airway procedures are exceeding useful in patients who are either unfit for intravenous sedation or who present significant anatomic challenges. Early experiences and preliminary studies confirm efficacy, safety, and patient tolerance comparable with or exceeding airway procedures performed in other settings.

REFERENCES

1. Whited RE. A prospective study of laryngotracheal sequelae in long-term intubation. Laryngoscope 1984;94:367–77.
2. Cummings CW. Cummings otolaryngology head & neck surgery. 4th edition. Philadelphia: Elsevier Mosby; 2005.
3. Arola MK, Inberg MV, Puhakka H. Tracheal stenosis after tracheostomy and after orotracheal cuffed intubation. Acta Chir Scand 1981;147:183–92.
4. Gaissert HA, Burns J. The compromised airway: tumors, strictures, and tracheomalacia. Surg Clin North Am 2010;90:1065–89.
5. Lorenz RR. Adult laryngotracheal stenosis: etiology and surgical management. Curr Opin Otolaryngol Head Neck Surg 2003;11:467–72.
6. Feinberg S, Lopez-Guerra G, Zeitels SM. Hypopharyngeal extrusion of 2.5 feet (76 cm) of polytetrafluoroethylene (Gore-Tex): initial laser-assisted office-based removal and micropharyngeal completion. Ann Otol Rhinol Laryngol 2010;119:573–7.
7. Lundgren R, Haggmark S, Reiz S. Hemodynamic effects of flexible fiberoptic bronchoscopy performed under topical anesthesia. Chest 1982;82:295–9.
8. Peacock AJ, Benson-Mitchell R, Godfrey R. Effect of fibreoptic bronchoscopy on pulmonary function. Thorax 1990;45:38–41.
9. McAlpine LG, Thomson NC. Lidocaine-induced bronchoconstriction in asthmatic patients. Relation to histamine airway responsiveness and effect of preservative. Chest 1989;96:1012–5.
10. Morris LG, Zeitler DM, Amin MR. Unsedated flexible fiberoptic bronchoscopy in the resident clinic: technique and patient satisfaction. Laryngoscope 2007;117:1159–62.

11. Webb AR, Fernando SS, Dalton HR, et al. Local anaesthesia for fibreoptic bronchoscopy: transcricoid injection or the "spray as you go" technique? Thorax 1990;45:474–7.
12. Rees CJ. In-office unsedated transnasal balloon dilation of the esophagus and trachea. Curr Opin Otolaryngol Head Neck Surg 2007;15:401–4.
13. Koufman JA, Rees CJ, Frazier WD, et al. Office-based laryngeal laser surgery: a review of 443 cases using three wavelengths. Otolaryngol Head Neck Surg 2007;137:146–51.
14. Amin MR, Simpson CB. Office evaluation of the tracheobronchial tree. Ear Nose Throat J 2004;83:10–2.
15. Lee KH, Ko GY, Song HY, et al. Benign tracheobronchial stenoses: long-term clinical experience with balloon dilation. J Vasc Interv Radiol 2002;13:909–14.
16. Kim JH, Shin JH, Song HY, et al. Tracheobronchial laceration after balloon dilation for benign strictures: incidence and clinical significance. Chest 2007;131:1114–7.
17. Daniel Knott P, Lorenz RR, Eliachar I, et al. Reconstruction of a tracheobronchial tree disruption with bovine pericardium. Interact Cardiovasc Thorac Surg 2004;3:554–6.
18. Kim JH, Shin JH, Shim TS, et al. Deep tracheal laceration after balloon dilation for benign tracheobronchial stenosis: case reports of two patients. Br J Radiol 2006;79:529–35.
19. Hogikyan ND. Transnasal endoscopic examination of the subglottis and trachea using topical anesthesia in the otolaryngology clinic. Laryngoscope 1999;109:1170–3.
20. Rees CJ, Halum SL, Wijewickrama RC, et al. Patient tolerance of in-office pulsed dye laser treatments to the upper aerodigestive tract. Otolaryngol Head Neck Surg 2006;134:1023–7.
21. Rosen CA, Amin MR, Sulica L, et al. Advances in office-based diagnosis and treatment in laryngology. Laryngoscope 2009;119(Suppl 2):S185–212.
22. Postma GN, Goins MR, Koufman JA. Office-based laser procedures for the upper aerodigestive tract: emerging technology. Ear Nose Throat J 2004;83:22–4.
23. Andrews BT, Graham SM, Ross AF, et al. Technique, utility, and safety of awake tracheoplasty using combined laser and balloon dilation. Laryngoscope 2007;117:2159–62.
24. Leventhal DD, Krebs E, Rosen MR. Flexible laser bronchoscopy for subglottic stenosis in the awake patient. Arch Otolaryngol Head Neck Surg 2009;135:467–71.
25. Rees CJ, Postma GN, Koufman JA. Cost savings of unsedated office-based laser surgery for laryngeal papillomas. Ann Otol Rhinol Laryngol 2007;116:45–8.
26. Kuo CY, Halum SL. Office-based laser surgery of the larynx: cost-effective treatment at the office's expense. Otolaryngol Head Neck Surg 2012;146:769–73.

Office-Based Laryngeal Procedures

Manish D. Shah, MD, MPhil[a], Michael M. Johns III, MD[b,*]

KEYWORDS

• Laryngeal • Larynx • Laryngeal surgery • Awake surgery

KEY POINTS

- Awake office-based laser procedures can be successfully used to treat a wide variety of laryngeal pathology including laryngeal papillomatosis, glottal leukoplakia and dysplasia, and Reinke's edema.
- Awake laser procedures are generally well-tolerated and safe with a very low incidence of complications.
- Appropriate flexible scope technology and laser selection is essential for safe and successful completion of these procedures.
- Laryngeal biopsies can be easily and safely performed in the office. Such biopsies have been shown to be as accurate as those done under general anesthesia in the operating room.

OFFICE-BASED LASER PROCEDURES

Nature of the Problem and Indications

The development of awake office-based laser procedures has dramatically changed the management of many laryngeal diseases. Such procedures offer several advantages for the patient and surgeon. From the patient perspective, awake procedures are significantly more convenient compared with procedures under general anesthesia or sedation. Patients may leave the hospital on their own and may even return to work the same day. Patient safety is further enhanced by avoiding the risks associated with general anesthesia. This is especially important for patients with significant comorbid medical conditions. Furthermore, certain laryngeal disease entities, such as glottal leukoplakia/dysplasia or papillomatosis, were once observed until severe enough to justify exposing the patient to the inconveniences and risks of general anesthesia. With the advent of effective awake procedures, these diseases can be treated as frequently as indicated by clinician concern and patient symptoms.

[a] Department of Otolaryngology Head & Neck Surgery, University of Toronto, 190 Elizabeth Street, Rm 3S-438, R. Fraser Elliott Building, Toronto, ON M5G 2N2 Canada; [b] Department of Otolaryngology Head & Neck Surgery, Emory University, 550 Peachtree Street NE, Suite 9-4400, Atlanta, GA 30308, USA

* Corresponding author.

E-mail address: michael.johns2@emory.edu

Otolaryngol Clin N Am 46 (2013) 75–84

http://dx.doi.org/10.1016/j.otc.2012.08.019 **oto.theclinics.com**

0030-6665/13/$ – see front matter

Studies have shown that awake laser treatment can be effective in appropriately selected cases of recurrent respiratory papillomatosis,[1–4] glottal leukoplakia/dysplasia,[4,5] and vascular lesions.[1,3,6] A variety of other lesions, such as vocal fold polyps, granulomas, Reinke edema, and laryngeal amyloidosis, have also been successfully treated.[2,3,7–10]

Preoperative Planning

Patients must be able to tolerate laryngeal visualization without an intense gag reflex. Patients who are not able to remain still for the duration of the procedure, such as those with cervical dystonias or severe head tremor, may be difficult to treat.[11] Anticoagulant or antiplatelet medications should be stopped before procedures if possible; however, in the experience of the authors and others,[11,12] complication rates are not higher in these patients even if they are unable to stop these medications.

Preparation and Patient Positioning

Most patients tolerate an awake laryngeal procedure; however, patient preparation is essential. The procedure must be clearly explained, including the abnormal sensations produced by topical anesthesia and the potential mild discomfort they may feel during the procedure. It is generally prudent to not attempt a procedure on a patient who seems too anxious to proceed. However, with adequate preprocedure explanations and coaching throughout, even very anxious patients tolerate an awake procedure.

For the purposes of this article, "office-based" implies that the patient is awake, with no or minimal sedation, sitting upright, and able to provide phonatory feedback. Often these procedures are done in hospital-based procedure rooms, such as endoscopy suites as opposed to an "office"; however, as long as there is adherence to these principles the potential advantages of these procedures are still realized.

Excellent laryngeal visualization is essential for successful awake laryngeal procedures. Rod-lens rigid endoscopes generally provide superior image quality compared with flexible fiberoptic endoscopes because of larger and more stable light-carrying fibers. However, the development of flexible endoscopes with a chip-based camera at the distal end of the scope has led to image quality that is almost equivalent to rigid rod-lens scopes.[13] Additionally, adequate anesthesia of the larynx and pharynx is critical to success. Details of this topic have been covered in detail by Wang and Simpson elsewhere in this issue.

Significant hemodynamic changes can be seen during these awake procedures. In a study of 31 patients who underwent close monitoring of their vital signs during their procedure, 23% of patients developed severe hypertension and 29% significant tachycardia.[14] Moreover, none of the patients reported or showed signs of an abnormal level of discomfort.[14] Others studies have reported that most patients tolerate awake procedures with minimal reported pain or discomfort.[15,16] This may suggest that patients are experiencing significant hemodynamic changes that do not correlate with subjective comfort levels. However, given the low incidence of reported complications with awake procedures, these changes likely do not pose a significant danger to most patients. Therefore, in general, it is the opinion of the authors that monitoring is not routinely indicated in patients who do not receive sedation. However, patients with medical comorbidities, such a severe cardiac or pulmonary disease, may benefit from pulse oximetry or blood pressure monitoring.

Procedural Approach

Laser selection

For awake office-based laser procedures, the laser must be deliverable through a fiber that can be passed through the working channel of a flexible endoscope (**Fig. 1**).

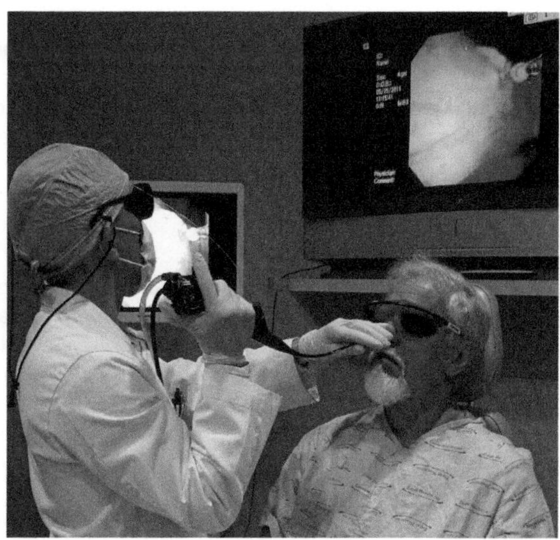

Fig. 1. Positioning of the surgeon and the patient for an awake office-based laser procedure.

The ideal laser for laryngeal surgery should possess the following properties: superficial penetration, minimal collateral thermal injury, and the ability to cut and coagulate.[17] The commonly described lasers for awake laryngeal surgery are discussed next.

The carbon dioxide (CO_2) laser has a wavelength of 10,600 nm and its target chromophore is water. The CO_2 laser was the first laser used for laryngeal surgery. There is a high concentration of water in laryngeal tissue, resulting in rapid dissipation of CO_2 laser energy without deeper penetration.[18] This allows the laser to cut with minimal collateral thermal injury. The CO_2 laser was initially developed for mirror reflected line-of-sight surgery, typically with an operating microscope. Its application to awake procedures was limited until the recently developed photonic bandgap fiber assembly (OmniGuide, Cambridge, MA), which allows it to be delivered through a flexible fiber.[18–20]

The thulium laser has a wavelength of 2013 nm and also has water as its target chromophore, resulting in similar properties to the CO_2 laser. However, its coagulation capabilities are superior, providing excellent hemostasis.[21] Furthermore, it can be delivered through a small flexible glass fiber, not requiring the expensive fiber required for flexible CO_2 laser delivery. Finally, the thulium laser can be used in contact and noncontact modes, a distinct advantage in awake laser surgery.

The pulse dye laser (PDL) has a wavelength of 585 nm. Unlike the CO_2 and thulium lasers, the chromophore is oxyhemoglobin. The proposed mechanism for the PDL is by damage to the walls of microvessels and surrounding perivascular tissue (photoangiolysis) because of its selectivity for oxyhemoglobin. This is thought to ablate a lesion's blood supply, leading to involution. However, it has also been shown to be effective for nonvascular lesions, suggesting that another mechanism of action is also at play. The PDL can also be used in contact or noncontact mode.[4]

The potassium titanyl phosphate (KTP) laser has a similar wavelength to the PDL at 532 nm and also shares oxyhemoglobin as the target chromophore. The wavelength of the KTP laser is more strongly absorbed by oxyhemoglobin and it has a longer pulse width compared with the PDL. It is theorized that this results in more effective intravascular coagulation and avoids vessel rupture and bleeding that can be encountered when using the PDL.[5,22] The KTP laser can be used in contact and noncontact modes, and either pulsed or continuous. This latter attribute is useful for hemostatic cutting. However, when used in this setting it has the potential to create more thermal injury when compared with the CO_2 or thulium lasers.[17]

Surgical technique

The surgical procedure is as follows:

- With the patient in a seated position and after application of appropriate anesthesia, a flexible scope is passed through the nasal cavity to visualize the larynx. Anesthesia can be applied to the larynx by the working channel of the scope or by other means (see the article by Wang and Simpson elsewhere in this issue).
- The laser fiber is then passed through the working channel of the scope until the tip of the fiber is visible 1 to 2 cm beyond the end of the scope. Laser settings vary by laser type; appropriate resources from the manufacturer and the literature should be consulted.
- Appropriate laser safety eyewear should be worn by the surgeon, patient, and other staff involved.
- The scope and fiber can then be manipulated and fired to allow either contact or noncontact treatment of the lesion.
- Sequential superficial blanching and gentle suctioning using the flexible scope allows for treatment of the lesion without undesired deep treatment of normal vocal fold tissue.

This technique exposes untreated disease below, which can be treated further to result in complete treatment of the lesion.

Postprocedure Care

Awake laser procedures are well-tolerated in patients who have received adequate topical anesthesia.[3–5,23] Most patients experience minimal pain, typically do not require any postoperative analgesia, and prefer the awake procedures to procedures done under general anesthetic.[15,23] Patients are typically discharged immediately after completion of the procedure and are instructed to take nothing by mouth for 30 to 45 minutes after the procedure because of the risk of aspiration secondary to laryngopharyngeal anesthesia.

Potential Complications

Complications rates are very low, with patient mild discomfort during the procedure being the most common complication.[2–5] It should be emphasized that appropriate laser safety precautions by the surgeon, patient, and other staff involved are essential. Vasovagal reactions can rarely occur,[24] but actual syncope can often be prevented if the prodromal symptoms are recognized. The procedure should be aborted and the patient placed in a reclined position. Koufman and colleagues[2] reported only 1 vasovagal reaction in 406 awake office-based laser procedures. Zeitels and colleagues[4] also reported 2 cases of minor epistaxis in a series of 82 awake laser procedures.

As with any laser laryngeal surgical procedure, there is the risk of inappropriate treatment of normal vocal fold tissue, which may result in scar or permanent worsening of the voice. Care must be taken to use appropriate laser energy settings and to follow the technique described previously to minimize the risk of such injury. Koufman and colleagues[2] did report one case of vocal fold hemorrhage. However, in two large published series there have been no reported cases of significant vocal fold scar or web formation.[2,3]

Reports of more serious complications are very rare. There has been one report of a laser fiber tip breaking and falling into the distal airway.[2] It was, however, easily retrieved in the awake patient. Mouadeb and Belafsky[3] reported one case of airway distress after treatment of Reinke edema that responded to medical management.

Rehabilitation and Recovery

Voice rest is typically recommended for 1 week. At this point in time, patients are reassessed and if healing is occurring appropriately, they may slowly return to full voice. Patients may require appropriate voice therapy postoperatively to deal with secondary functional voice problems.

Outcomes and Clinical Results in the Literature

Papilloma

The selectivity of the PDL and KTP laser for oxyhemoglobin, combined with the abundant vascular supply to papillomas, has made these lasers very popular in treatment recurrent respiratory papillomas in the office setting (**Figs. 2** and **3**). Numerous studies have shown that these lasers provide effective and safe treatment for papillomas.[1–4] Thulium and flexible CO_2 lasers have also been used for awake treatment of papillomas.[2,21] Patients presenting with a new diagnosis of recurrent respiratory papillomas should be treated for the first time under general anesthetic, allowing for disease mapping and tissue biopsies. Subsequent procedures can be done in the office setting depending on the amount and extent of disease. The amount of disease that can be treated awake depends on patient tolerance and surgeon experience (see **Figs. 2** and **3**).

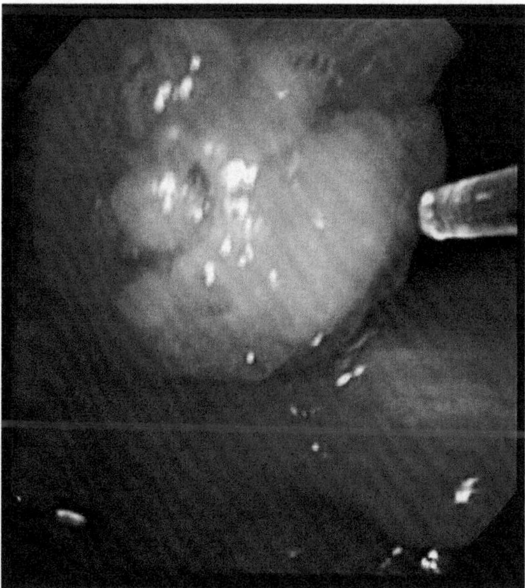

Fig. 2. The pulsed KTP laser being used to treat recurrent respiratory papillomas of the true vocal folds in noncontact mode. The superficial papilloma (*notice the blanched color*) is treated while avoiding significant bleeding.

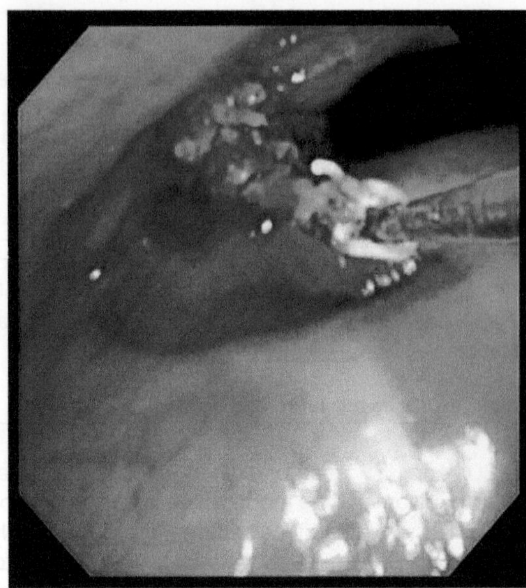

Fig. 3. The pulsed KTP laser is used to treat papillomas on the true vocal folds in contact mode. The treated superficial papilloma is removed, permitting further treatment of deeper papilloma.

Glottal leuokplakia/dysplasia

There are a variety of management options for patients with glottal leukoplakia or dysplasia. These include biopsy and observation, phonomicrosurgical excision, and laser resection or ablation. Recurrent or persistent glottal disease is not uncommon and this poses a dilemma. The surgeon must weight the negative consequences of repeated general anesthesia and vocal fold surgery against the risks of disease progression with observation alone. Awake laser treatment provides the surgeon and patient a low-morbidity option in this situation.[4,5] Because of their presumed photoangiolytic properties, the PDL and KTP laser have gained popularity in treating the microcirculatory supply of these lesions. Numerous studies support their efficacy in causing regression of visible disease.[1–5]

Vascular lesions

Vascular ectasias and varices can require surgical treatment because they can impair the normal vibratory pattern of the vocal fold and they can rupture, causing vocal fold hemorrhage. Again, because of the presumed photoangiolytic properties of the PDL and KTP laser, these have been successful in treating such lesions.[1,3,6]

Other laryngeal pathology

A variety of other lesions have been treated with mixed success using awake laser procedures, including vocal fold polyps, granulomas, Reinke edema, and laryngeal amyloidosis.[2,3,7–10]

LARYNGOPHARYNGEAL BIOPSY, PANENDOSCOPY, AND TUMOR STAGING

Nature of the Problem and Indications

Traditionally, patients with laryngeal lesions suspicious for premalignancy or malignancy underwent diagnostic laryngoscopy and biopsy in the operating room under general anesthesia. This has the obvious disadvantages of delaying the diagnosis while waiting for scheduled operating room time, the risks of general anesthesia, and the risks of direct laryngoscopy (eg, dental injury). Using awake office-based techniques, most laryngeal lesions can be safely biopsied in an office-based setting.

Preoperative Planning, Preparation, and Patient Positioning

The issues here are similar to those discussed previously for office-based laser procedures.

Procedural Approach

There are two techniques that can be used to conduct office-based laryngeal biopsies: peroral technique or by a flexible endoscope.

Peroral biopsies can be done with a rigid scope and a long curved biopsy forceps (**Fig. 4**) after appropriate topical anesthesia of the larynx. The patient holds on to their tongue while the surgeon directs the scope and biopsy forceps. Alternatively, the larynx can be viewed with a flexible scope held by and assistant while the surgeon holds the patient's tongue and directs the biopsy forceps through the oral cavity. The peroral technique, however, can be difficult to perform and is not well tolerated by all patients.

The other technique for biopsies involves using a flexible endoscope with a working channel through which a small flexible biopsy forceps can be passed. This technique is generally better tolerated by most patients in the experience of the authors. The scope is advanced to a position with the lesion of interest in view and a 1.8-mm flexible cup biopsy forceps is passed through the working channel by an assistant until visible 1 to 2 cm beyond the tip of the scope. The forceps are then opened and the scope is advanced until the forceps come into contact with the lesion (**Fig. 5**). The forceps are then closed and removed from the scope. The scope can be left in place and multiple biopsies can be taken. This is often advisable as false-negative results are possible because of the small size of the biopsy forceps.

Immediate Postprocedural Care

Awake laryngeal biopsies are typically well-tolerated and most patients experience minimal or no pain. Patients are typically discharged immediately following the procedures. Patients must be instructed to take nothing by mouth for 30 to 45 minutes after the procedure because of the risk of aspiration secondary to laryngopharyngeal anesthesia.

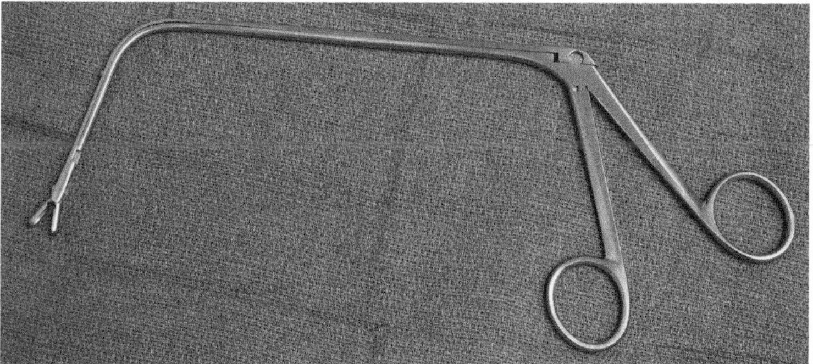

Fig. 4. Curved biopsy forceps for peroral laryngeal biopsies.

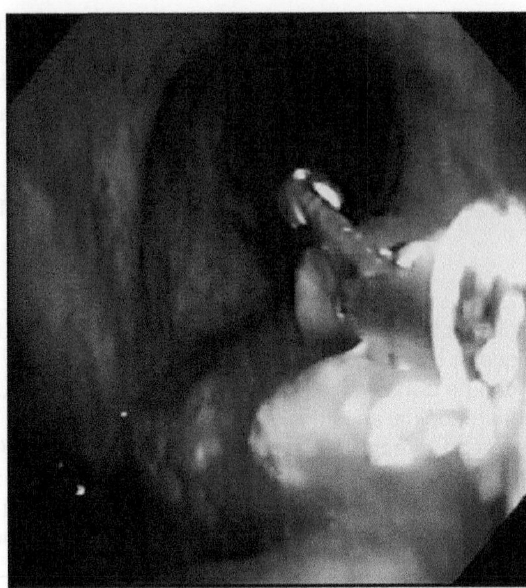

Fig. 5. A true vocal fold lesion being biopsied using a flexible biopsy forceps passed through the working channel of a flexible scope.

Potential Complications

As with any awake laryngeal procedure, complications related to topical anesthesia are possible. Vasovagal reactions do occur, but are rare.[24] A small amount of bleeding is normal and is almost always self-limited. Although the biopsy forceps are quite small in caliber, it is possible to traumatize normal vocal fold tissue if excessively deep biopsies are taken. To avoid any potentially deleterious consequences, biopsies should be taken from a nonphonatory surface of the vocal fold where possible.

Rehabilitation and Recovery

Healing after superficial laryngeal biopsies generally takes places very quickly and voice rest is not typically required after the procedure.

Outcomes and Clinical Results in the Literature

Detailed indirect laryngoscopy in the office setting, along with biopsies, can provide an equal degree of diagnostic information when compared with direct laryngoscopy and biopsies in the operating room.[25] Furthermore, the ability to conduct biopsies, along with transnasal esophagoscopy and awake bronchscopy, allows for awake panendoscopy and tumor staging to be done in the office setting. This has been demonstrated to be as accurate as operative staging under general anesthesia.[26] Transnasal esophagoscopy and airway assessment are discussed further elsewhere in this issue (see the articles by Bush and Postma, and Shah and Johns).

SUMMARY

Awake office-based laryngeal procedures are well-tolerated, safe, and can be used to treat a wide variety of laryngeal pathology. Technologic advancements have allowed for these procedures to flourish and develop. Appropriate surgeon training and experience, along with careful patient selection and preparation, is essential to maximize success and reduce the incidence of complications.

REFERENCES

1. Burns JA, Friedman AD, Lutch MJ, et al. Value and utility of 532 nanometre pulse potassium-titanyl-phosphate laser in endoscopic laryngeal surgery. J Laryngol Otol 2010;124:407–11.
2. Koufman JA, Rees CJ, Frazier WD, et al. Office-based laryngeal laser surgery: a review of 443 cases using three wavelengths. Otolaryngol Head Neck Surg 2007;137:146–51.
3. Mouadeb DA, Belafsky PC. In-office laryngeal surgery with the 585nm pulsed dye laser (PDL). Otolaryngol Head Neck Surg 2007;137:477–81.
4. Zeitels SM, Franco RA Jr, Dailey SH, et al. Office-based treatment of glottal dysplasia and papillomatosis with the 585-nm pulsed dye laser and local anesthesia. Ann Otol Rhinol Laryngol 2004;113:265–76.
5. Zeitels SM, Akst LM, Burns JA, et al. Office-based 532-nm pulsed KTP laser treatment of glottal papillomatosis and dysplasia. Ann Otol Rhinol Laryngol 2006;115: 679–85.
6. Zeitels SM, Akst LM, Burns JA, et al. Pulsed angiolytic laser treatment of ectasias and varices in singers. Ann Otol Rhinol Laryngol 2006;115:571–80.
7. Clyne SB, Halum SL, Koufman JA, et al. Pulsed dye laser treatment of laryngeal granulomas. Ann Otol Rhinol Laryngol 2005;114:198–201.
8. Ivey CM, Woo P, Altman KW, et al. Office pulsed dye laser treatment for benign laryngeal vascular polyps: a preliminary study. Ann Otol Rhinol Laryngol 2008; 117:353–8.
9. Kim HT, Auo HJ. Office-based 585 nm pulsed dye laser treatment for vocal polyps. Acta Otolaryngol 2008;128:1043–7.
10. Mallur PS, Tajudeen BA, Aaronson N, et al. Quantification of benign lesion regression as a function of 532-nm pulsed potassium titanyl phosphate laser parameter selection. Laryngoscope 2011;121:590–5.
11. Simpson CB, Amin MR, Postma GN. Topical anesthesia of the airway and esophagus. Ear Nose Throat J 2004;83(7 Suppl 2):2–5.
12. Bastian R, Delsupehe K. Indirect larynx and pharynx surgery: a replacement for direct laryngoscopy. Laryngoscope 1996;106:1280–6.
13. Eller R, Ginsburg M, Lurie D, et al. Flexible laryngoscopy: a comparison of fiber optic and distal chip technologies. Part 1: vocal fold masses. J Voice 2008;22:746–50.
14. Yung KC, Courey MS. The effect of office-based flexible endoscopic surgery on hemodynamic stability. Laryngoscope 2010;120:2231–6.
15. Rees CJ, Halum SL, Wijewickrama RC, et al. Patient tolerance of in-office pulsed dye laser treatments to the upper aerodigestive tract. Otolaryngol Head Neck Surg 2006;134:1023–7.
16. Postma GN, Cohen JT, Belafsky PC, et al. Transnasal esophagoscopy: revisited (over 700 consecutive cases). Laryngoscope 2005;115:321–3.
17. Rosen CA, Amin MR, Sulica L, et al. Advances in office-based diagnosis and treatment in laryngology. Laryngoscope 2009;119(S2):S185–212.
18. Devaiah AK, Shapshay SM, Desai U, et al. Surgical utility of a new carbon dioxide laser fiber: functional and histological study. Laryngoscope 2005;115:1463–8.
19. Shurgalin M, Anastassiou C. A new modality for minimally invasive CO2 laser surgery: flexible hollow-core photonic bandgap fibers. Biomed Instrum Technol 2008;42:318–25.

20. Zeitels SM, Kobler JB, Heaton JT, et al. Carbon dioxide laser fiber for laryngeal cancer surgery. Ann Otol Rhinol Laryngol 2006;115:535–41.
21. Zeitels SM, Burns JA, Akst LM, et al. Office-based and microlaryngeal applications of a fiber-based thulium laser. Ann Otol Rhinol Laryngol 2006;115:891–6.
22. Broadhurst MS, Akst LM, Burns JA, et al. Effects of 532 nm pulsed-KTP laser parameters on vessel ablation in the avian chorioallantoic membrane: implications for vocal fold mucosa. Laryngoscope 2007;117:220–5.
23. Young VN, Smith LJ, Sulica L, et al. Patient tolerance of awake, in-office laryngeal procedures: a multi-institutional perspective. Laryngoscope 2012;122:315–21.
24. Sulica L, Blitzer A. Anesthesia for laryngeal surgery in the office. Laryngoscope 2000;100(10 pt 1):1777–9.
25. Bastian RW, Collins SL, Kaniff T, et al. Indirect videolaryngoscopy versus direct endoscopy for larynx and pharynx cancer staging. Toward elimination of preliminary direct laryngoscopy. Ann Otol Rhinol Laryngol 1989;98:693–8.
26. Postma GN, Bach KK, Belafsky PC, et al. The role of transnasal esophagoscopy in head and neck oncology. Laryngoscope 2002;112:2242–3.

Office-Based Laryngeal Injections

Pavan S. Mallur, MD[a,b], Clark A. Rosen, MD[c,*]

KEYWORDS

• Larynx • Laryngeal injections • Vocal fold injection • Ambulatory surgery
• Surgical procedures

KEY POINTS

- Office-based vocal fold injection (VFI) is emerging as the standard of care for the treatment of glottal incompetence in select patients.
- Successful office-based VFI is predicated on systematic planning, and requires proper patient selection, surgeon and staff familiarity, specialized equipment, and a procedural assistant who is accomplished in flexible laryngoscopy.
- The principal advantages of office-based VFI are avoidance of general anesthesia, patient convenience, and real-time assessment of injection results and voice outcome.

OVERVIEW

Deep Vocal Fold Injection

Deep vocal fold injection (VFI) functions to correct glottal incompetence from various causes. Materials injected into the lateral aspect of the thyroarytenoid/lateral cricoarytenoid muscle complex (medial aspect of the paraglottic space) result in an augmented and/or medially displaced vocal fold. Cadaveric studies suggest that increased free-edge height and medial rotation and displacement of the arytenoid may be added benefits, although these subtle effects have not been substantiated in live subjects with residual motion or synkinetic tone.[1,2] Deep VFI is most commonly used to address dysphonia and dysphagia associated with vocal fold immobility or paralysis. Advances in the safety profile of injection materials have broadened the indications to include glottal insufficiency arising from vocal fold hypomobility or paresis, vocal fold atrophy, and vocal fold scar or sulcus vocalis.[3,4]

Current nomenclature classifies deep VFI into temporary, trial, or permanent/durable, based on duration of material biointegration and indication.

Temporary VFI is most commonly used to restore glottal competence in patients with an acute vocal fold paralysis or paresis with expectant or unknown recovery.

[a] Department of Otology and Laryngology, Harvard Medical School, 234 Charles Street, Boston, MA 02115, USA; [b] Department of Surgery, Beth Israel Deaconess Medical Center, 110 Francis Street, Suite 6E, Boston, MA 02115, USA; [c] Department of Otolaryngology, University of Pittsburgh Voice Center, University of Pittsburgh School of Medicine, 1400 Locust Street, Building B, Suite 11500, Pittsburgh, PA 15219, USA
* Corresponding author.
E-mail address: rosenca@upmc.edu

Otolaryngol Clin N Am 46 (2013) 85–100
http://dx.doi.org/10.1016/j.otc.2012.08.020 oto.theclinics.com

In certain clinical scenarios it is unclear whether vocal fold augmentation will result in improved voice, as is common with vocal fold atrophy, scar, and sulcus vocalis. In these instances, patients may undergo a trial injection to determine if, and to what extent, augmentation will provide symptomatic improvement.[5]

Permanent/durable VFI is used to treat glottal incompetence that is long-standing or paralysis/paresis that has a poor prognosis for recovery. In addition, permanent VFI may be used after a positive result with trial VFI.[5]

Materials for deep VFI are typically classified based on the duration of biointegration or, more practically, duration of efficacy.

The durable material most commonly used for office-based VFI is calcium hydroxylapatite (Radiesse Voice). Office-based autologous fat injection is not routinely performed secondary to the need for subcutaneous harvest and requirement of a large-bore needle for injection.

Temporary injection materials used in-office include collagen-based products (Cymetra), hyaluronic acid (Restylane, Hyalaform), and carboxymethylcellulose (Radiesse Voice Gel).

Clinically, the material's expected duration of efficacy guides selection, and pragmatically, ease of preparation and delivery may also factor into surgeon preference. Several available materials are provided ready-to-use in a self-contained delivery system, increasing convenience and decreasing preparation time. Materials also vary in biocompatibility and viscoelastic properties, and although this may guide surgeon selection, systematic comparison of voice outcomes with modern materials has not been reported to date.

Superficial Vocal Fold Injection

Superficial VFI is a distinct office-based injection that targets the subepithelial space of the vocal fold. With this technique, the subepithelial space is injected with biomaterials to replace the lamina propria or inflammatory modulators to promote scar remodeling. It is indicated for vocal fold scar and lamina propria deficits, with the goal of improving vibratory abnormalities and medial edge height, rather than providing global augmentation or medialization. The limited materials applicable for superficial VFI have been used sparingly and have not been studied extensively. Superficial saline infusion has been described as a diagnostic means of assessing the extent of tethered scar.[6] Temporary lamina propria replacements include collagen.[7] In clinical practice, corticosteroid injection is the most commonly used scar modulator.[8] Though still experimental, promising small-scale trials have examined superficial VFI with autologous fibroblasts to promote lamina propria regeneration.[9]

VFI as Viable Alternative to Microsuspension or Direct Laryngoscopy

Several factors have established office-based VFI as a viable alternative to microsuspension or direct laryngoscopy VFI. Pointing to the popularity of this technique, a recent multi-institutional review revealed that VFI was performed equally often in the office as in the operating room.[3] Office-based VFI has the distinct advantage of allowing real-time assessment of injection results and voice outcome during the procedure. Inherent risks of general anesthesia can be avoided, especially in patients with medical comorbidities. In addition, office-based VFI does not carry the risks associated with oral and pharyngeal trauma from rigid endoscopy. Voice outcomes are comparable between the two settings, and complications are typically minor and self-resolving.[9,10] Patient preference may play a role as well. Patients avoid preoperative workup, have the procedure completed in 1-2 hours, and are able to resume daily activities immediately. Finally, with a national drive toward reducing health care spending, the dramatic cost reduction of VFI in the office in comparison with an operating-room procedure should not be ignored.[9]

Office-based VFI may be performed through several approaches:

- Peroral
- Percutaneous
- Transcricothyroid and transthyroid cartilage
- Transnasal endoscopic

The peroral approach uses a curved needle directed through the oral cavity and oropharynx toward the vocal folds.

Percutaneous VFI techniques are performed by passing the injection needle into the vocal fold via a transcricothyroid membrane, transthyroid cartilage, or transthyrohyoid membrane route.

With the transcricothyroid and transthyroid cartilage approaches, the needle is passed through the skin and takes an entirely submucosal or "blind" path to the vocal fold. The transthyrohyoid approach is distinct from the other percutaneous approaches in that the needle tip takes a visualized, intraluminal path to the vocal fold after insertion through the thyrohyoid membrane.

The transnasal endoscopic approach uses a 23- or 25-gauge flexible needle delivered through the working channel of a flexible laryngoscope, and may require a high-pressure injection device, depending on the material of choice. In most cases of the above approaches, an assistant provides visualization with a distal-chip flexible laryngoscope for confirmation of needle placement and observation of injection results.

Some have also described peroral VFI using a 70° rigid telescope for visualization. Each approach has advantages and disadvantages, and selection is often based on surgeon familiarity and experience. Certain patient factors, such as oropharyngeal or supraglottic anatomy, strong gag reflex, and external neck anatomy may preclude one or more approaches. Thus the laryngologist is well served by being facile with at least several of the above-described approaches.

PREOPERATIVE PLANNING

Patient's Mental Faculties

Initial screening for office-based injection should begin with assessment of the candidate's mental faculties. A patient should be cooperative, able to follow commands appropriately, and be able to sit upright without assistance. To this end, a proper candidate for office-based injection should have relatively intact cognition; this excludes, with exception, very young children and patients with deficits of mental status.

Anxiety may play a large factor in patient selection, as even the patient with the best intentions may become uncooperative if extremely anxious. Anxiety should be assessed during the preprocedural visit, and if needed the surgeon may prescribe an oral benzodiazepine, such as diazepam 1 mg or alprazolam 0.25 mg or 0.5 mg, to be taken by the patient several hours before the procedure. If an oral benzodiazepine is prescribed, the patient should provide written consent for the VFI before taking this, and should not drive on the day of the procedure. Anxiety levels toward in-office procedures have been shown not to change procedure completion rates.[11] However, these results likely have a selection bias, as patients who are able to overcome anxiety are more likely to be selected for office-based procedures.

Patient's Physical and Anatomic Aspects

The second consideration in screening for office-based VFI should be the physical and anatomic aspects of the candidate. Adequate nasal patency and presence of septal deflections should be assessed, as most office-based VFIs are performed with a larger-caliber working-channel flexible laryngoscope. Although this is rarely a limiting factor, the occasional patient will have a nasal passage that cannot accommodate the larger laryngoscope. For planned peroral VFI, the oropharynx and supraglottis should be assessed to ensure that large base of tongue, elongated soft palate, redundant tonsil pillars, retroflexed epiglottis, and occasionally anterior cervical spine osteophytes will not physically impede the needle from reaching the larynx. Especially important is a candidate's gag reflex; a strong gag reflex may not be overcome even after adequate anesthesia, which can prevent successful peroral VFI. Poor visualization, attributed to overhanging arytenoid cartilage or false vocal fold abnormalities, accounts for a small percentage of procedure failures.[11,12] For planned percutaneous VFI, the surgeon must ensure that the laryngeal cartilages can be readily palpated and used as surface landmarks; patients with large necks or previous neck surgery may potentially be excluded from these approaches. Radiation to the larynx is not a contraindication in itself, and percutaneous VFI in such patients has been proved to be safe, although it may be more challenging.[13]

Anticoagulation status should be noted, although office-based VFI has been shown to be safe in patients taking anticoagulation medication. Evidence points away from airway obstruction or permanent sequelae secondary to hemorrhage during office-based VFI. Paraglottic hematoma and vocal fold hemorrhage have been reported, although the relation to anticoagulation is not consistent.[12] In patients taking warfarin, it is prudent to check preprocedural international normalized ratio to ensure the level is not supratherapeutic. In most instances patients taking warfarin, aspirin, clopidogrel, or other anticoagulants/antiplatelets can be continued on these medications safely, as the risks of stopping them may be greater than the risks attributed to office-based VFI.

High Completion Rates are Typical

Overall, tolerance for office-based VFI is very good, highlighted by a high completion rate of VFI in the literature. In a recent multi-institutional prospective study, 93% of patients were able to complete a first-choice approach for office-based VFI. Of the 7% requiring a second or third approach, 87.5% successfully completed the injection.[11] Because of such an eventuality, it is helpful if the surgeon is familiar with more than one technique for office-based VFI. Patient tolerance factors attributed to failure include excess secretions, inability to suppress gag reflex, and vasovagal syncope, although these were found in a minority of patients overall.[11,12]

PREPARATION AND PATIENT POSITIONING

Preparation for office-based VFI begins with a detailed instruction set for the patient. Separate from informed consent, providing the patient with a step-by-step list of the pending procedure allows the patient to anticipate instructions during the procedure and increases the ability to cooperate. This instruction may alleviate patient anxiety regarding an unfamiliar procedure, and is often referred to as "verbal anesthesia." (L. Sulica, personal communication, 2006).

Anesthesia for office-based VFI follows protocols that are covered in the article by Wang and Simpson elsewhere in this issue. In brief, nasal anesthesia is achieved by placing pledgets soaked with a 1:1 mixture of phenylephrine and 2% tetracaine. Some advocate global oropharyngeal and laryngeal anesthetic with a 4% lidocaine nebulization; this is particularly useful for peroral injections, and is helpful, though not universally required, for percutaneous approaches. With percutaneous approaches, the subcutaneous tissue overlying the landmark of interest is injected with 1% lidocaine with 1:100,000 epinephrine. An additional 4% lidocaine is given during a laryngeal gargle on an as-needed basis. This gargle may be achieved via a drip catheter through the working channel of a flexible laryngoscope, via an Abraham cannula placed perorally, or through the thyrohyoid membrane, if the thyrohyoid approach is planned.

The position of the patient, surgeon, assistant, and equipment remains fairly consistent across the approaches.

- The patient is seated upright.
- Waist and neck flexion with head extension, the so-called sniffing position, may facilitate views of the larynx; patient comfort must be taken into account, although most will be able to tolerate this positioning.
- Patients may turn their head to the left or right, to facilitate views of the right and left vocal fold, respectively.
- Patients may also be given a connected Yankaur suction or emesis basin ahead of time, as secretions tend to increase dramatically after laryngeal anesthesia.
- During peroral and thyrohyoid injection, the surgeon stands to the right of the patient and slightly anterior, while the assistant operating the flexible laryngoscope stands to the left and slightly anterior (**Fig. 1**).
- The video tower and screen are usually placed left and posterior of the patient. A screen mounted on articulating arms may be brought closer and angled toward the surgeon's line of view. An additional screen placed to the right and posterior of the patient can be angled toward the assistant's line of view (see **Fig. 1**).
- A small Mayo stand with the required instruments and injection material may be placed to the front or left of the surgeon (see **Fig. 1**).
- An additional assistant to hand the surgeon instrumentation is helpful, but not absolutely required.

Exceptions to this positioning occur during the transcricothyroid and transthyroid cartilage approaches.

- Needle insertion in these cases is based on the laterality of the injection, as the needle takes a completely submucosal course toward the vocal fold.

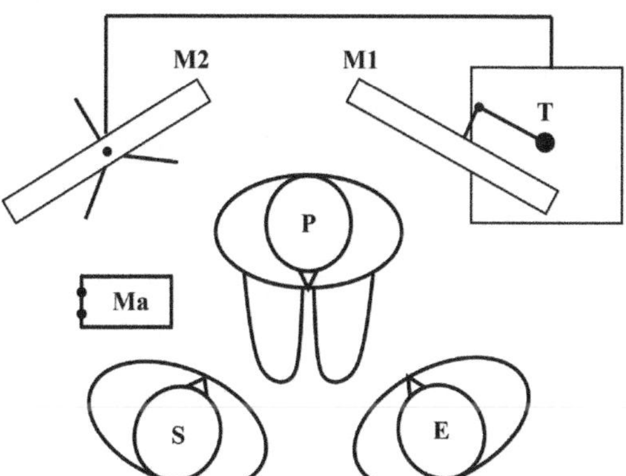

Fig. 1. The spatial orientation of the surgeon, assistant, patient, and equipment during in-office vocal fold injection. The surgeon (S) stands in front and to the right of the patient (P), while the endoscopist (E) stands in front and to the left. The video tower (T) hosts a monitor (M1) angled toward the surgeon, while a second, optional monitor (M2) faces the endoscopist. A small Mayo stand (Ma) is helpful to keep the injection needle and material in close proximity to the surgeon.

- The surgeon may stand to the left or right of the patient for left or right VFI, respectively.
- The assistant operating the flexible laryngoscope will alternate sides, moving to the opposite side of the surgeon as needed.
- Alternatively, some surgeons may prefer to remain to the right of the patient regardless of the side to be injected.

Equipment and material preparation are predicated on the route of injection and choice of injection material. All equipment should be readily available before the start of the procedure. Surgeons may opt to open the injection material only when they are sure the patient can tolerate the procedure. Although this causes minor delay in injection once adequate anesthesia has been achieved, it is usually limited and does not impede the actual injection.

With regard to materials, carboxymethylcellulose (Radiesse Voice Gel; Merz Aesthetics Inc, San Mateo, CA), hyaluronic acid (Restylane; Medicis Aesthetics Inc, Scottsdale, AZ; and Hyalform; INAMED Aesthetics Inc, Irvine, CA), and calcium hydroxylapatite (Radiesse Voice; Merz Aesthetics Inc, San Mateo, CA) are supplied as commercially available preparations and come ready-to-use in self-contained syringes. Of note, calcium hydroxylapatite has a high viscosity and may require gentle warming in a water bath or in a pant pocket to facilitate injection. Collagen-based products (Cymetra; Lifecell Corp, Branchburg, NJ) should be prepared ahead of time, as they require reconstitution in a process that takes several minutes. Methylprednisone for superficial VFI is provided reconstituted, but needs to be drawn into an appropriate syringe. Higher concentrations of methylprednisone (40 mg/mL) may settle into particulate and carrier layers, requiring shaking or physical mixing before use. Once materials are ready, injection needles should be primed to the needle tip to avoid injection of air.

PROCEDURAL APPROACH

Peroral Vocal Fold Injection

The peroral route uses a direct approach for VFI.

- After appropriate laryngeal anesthesia, the patient is positioned upright, with the neck flexed and head slightly extended.
- The patient protrudes the tongue and holds it externally with gauze.
- With the flexible laryngoscope in the oropharynx, the trajectory from oropharynx to vocal folds is estimated using a malleable Abraham catheter; this is typically a 90° path, although it may vary from patient to patient.
- Injection needles commonly used are the 27-gauge curved orotracheal injector device (Medtronic Xomed, Jackson, FL) or the 24-gauge malleable injection needle (Merz Aesthetics Inc, San Mateo, CA). The latter is easily bent to suit the individual patient's anatomy.
- The flexible laryngoscope is positioned at the level of the soft palate as the curved needle is introduced horizontally into the oropharynx (**Fig. 2**A).
- Once the needle tip is visualized endoscopically, the surgeon turns the needle 90° toward a vertical orientation and advances past the epiglottis.
- The assistant should advance the laryngoscope opposite the vocal fold to be injected: if the left vocal fold is to be injected, the laryngoscope should remain to the right of the injection needle, and vice versa for the right vocal fold (**Fig. 2**B). This action prevents physical interference and allows an unobstructed view of the target vocal fold.[14]

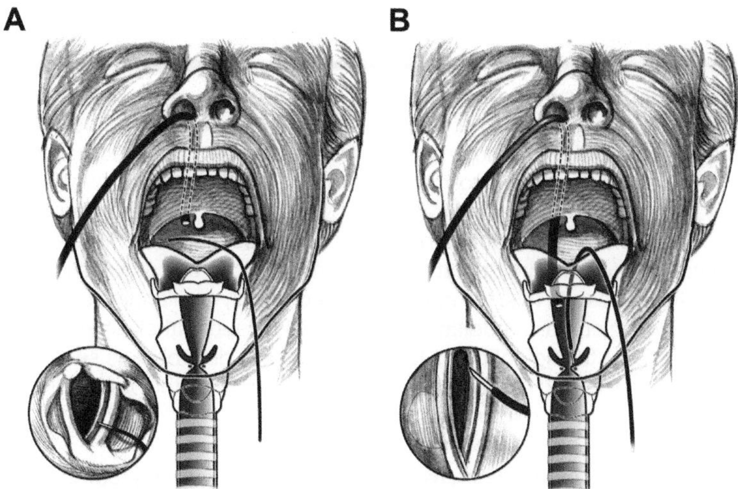

Fig. 2. Needle trajectory during peroral in-office vocal fold injection. (*A*) Horizontal entry of the needle with the laryngoscope placed at the level of the soft palate. (*B*) Laryngoscope advanced opposite the vocal fold to be injected, avoiding physical interference with the injection needle. (*From* Mallur PS, Rosen CA. Techniques for the laryngology assistant: providing optimal visualization. Oper Techniques Otolaryngol 2012;25:197–202; with permission.)

- The target for needle insertion should initially be the posterior membranous vocal fold, lateral to the vocal process; this should place the needle into the lateral aspect of the thyroarytenoid muscle/medial aspect of the paraglottic space.
- Once the needle is inserted, the laryngoscope is positioned to provide visualization of the entire vocal fold, especially the superior surface, free edge, and infraglottic aspects. Material injection should proceed at this point. If subglottic augmentation is seen initially, the needle should be withdrawn slightly and injection should resume. Withdrawing the needle excessively may inadvertently lead to a subepithelial location of the needle tip and unintended superficial injection into the Reinke space.
- If additional augmentation is needed, the needle is withdrawn and reinserted just lateral to the midmembranous portion of the thyroarytenoid muscle (mid-vocal fold).
- Most materials require a small amount of overinjection (0.1–0.2 mL) to compensate for minor material extrusion and resorption of aqueous carriers.
- The vocal fold is injected until a slight convexity of the free edge is achieved and/or improvement in voice with slight strain is noted. Initial voice strain is common immediately after a correctly performed injection.

Peroral VFI can also be performed with a 70° or 90° rigid telescope with the surgeon holding both the telescope and injection needle. As previously described, the patient assumes the "sniffing position" and retracts his or her own tongue.

- A right-handed surgeon typically holds the telescope in the left hand and the injection needle in the right.
- The telescope is used to visualize the larynx, and the injection needle is introduced into the oral cavity and advanced past the oropharynx.
- The surgeon may angle the telescope or alter the position for optimal visualization, and the injection proceeds as previously described.

This approach is a viable alternative to flexible laryngoscopy, as it gives the surgeon control of both visualization and injection, which may be especially useful if distal-chip laryngoscopes or procedural assistants to drive flexible laryngoscopy are not available.

Advantages and disadvantages of peroral approach

There are several advantages and disadvantages of the peroral approach. The principal advantages are the excellent needle visualization and the precision offered by watching the needle insertion into the vocal fold. The surgeon has excellent control of range of motion and can alter the trajectory by millimeters to change the target location of the vocal fold. This control is beneficial when focal deficits require multiple or specific injection sites for augmentation, as seen with scar, sulcus vocalis, or atrophy with focal deficits. Despite this, the approach is technically challenging to navigate and has a steep learning curve. In addition, the potential for subepithelial hemorrhage may be higher in patients taking anticoagulation. The largest drawback is seen in patients with a strong gag reflex; patients who cannot suppress the gag reflex despite adequate anesthesia may not tolerate peroral VFI.

Percutaneous Vocal Fold Injection (Transcricothyroid and Transthyroid Cartilage)

The transcricothyroid membrane approach is a widely used percutaneous route that can use an entirely submucosal path of the needle.

- The procedure starts with the patient in neutral neck position and slight head extension.
- Anesthetic is provided as previously described, and the skin is cleaned.
- Flexible laryngoscopy can proceed directly toward a close, unobstructed view of the vocal folds.
- To estimate the level of the vocal folds, the thyroid ala and cricothyroid membrane are palpated while viewing endoscopically for direct indentation of the infraglottis.
- A 25-gauge or 23-gauge needle is inserted just below the inferior border of the thyroid cartilage, 5 to 7 mm lateral to midline, and advanced 3 to 4 mm perpendicular to the thyroid ala (**Fig. 3**A).

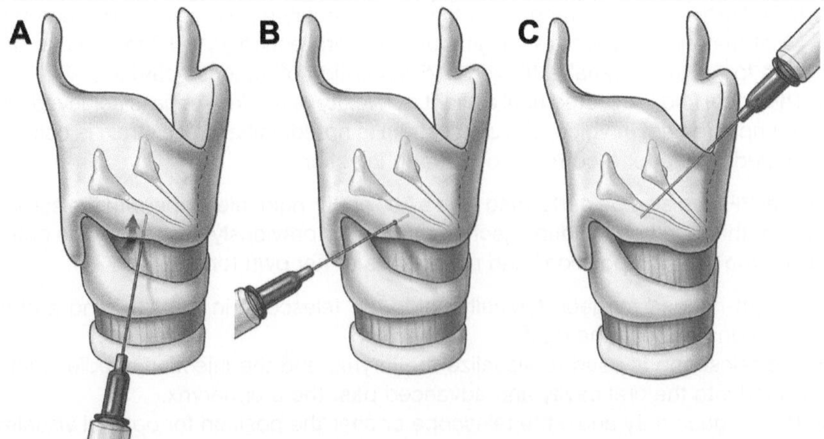

Fig. 3. (*A*) Transcricothyroid, (*B*) transthyroid cartilage, and (*C*) transthyrohyoid membrane approaches to vocal fold injection. (*From* Rosen CA, Simpson CB. Operative Techniques in Laryngology. Heidelberg: Springer, 2008; with permission.)

- The needle is then directed cephalad and passed slowly back and forth to look for transmitted motion and confirm placement at the vertical level of the vocal fold (see **Fig. 3**A).
- The needle should be advanced slowly to avoid mucosal perforation, and it should not be tenting the mucosa focally, which would indicate a subepithelial location.
- Injection should proceed while observing endoscopically for augmentation until the desired augmentation and voice results are achieved.

Similarly, the transthyroid cartilage approach uses a submucosal path.

- A 24-gauge or 25-gauge needle is inserted 3 to 5 mm above the lower border of the thyroid cartilage, 6 to 12 mm from the midline, and passed gently through the cartilage at a perpendicular trajectory (**Fig. 3**B).
- Once through cartilage, advancing the needle medially with gentle pressure transmits motion to the vocal fold, and allows the surgeon to estimate the location of the needle tip. Inadvertent mucosal perforation may occur with excessive medial pressure.
- Obstruction of the needle with cartilage may be overcome with incremental pressure applied to the plunger; excessive pressure during this step may lead to over-injection of material. This technique is optimal for younger patients without extensively calcified cartilage.

A trocar-based injection device has been made to assist transthyroid cartilage VFI (Casiano Needle; Medtronic Inc, Jacksonville, FL).

Advantages and disadvantages of transcricothyroid and transthyroid cartilage approach

Both the transcricothyroid and transthyroid cartilage VFI are useful as approaches that do not require a directly visualized pathway. In patients with favorable anatomy and easily palpated landmarks, the trajectory is predictable, easily controlled, and readily reproducible from patient to patient. The percutaneous approaches have the advantage of avoiding oropharyngeal stimulation in patients with strong gag reflexes that would preclude a peroral VFI. However, needle localization is blind and, therefore, less precise. Because of this, focal augmentation becomes more challenging and in some cases impossible with this technique. With the transthyroid cartilage approach, the injection needle is prone to obstruction, and in elderly patients may not be possible without a large-bore needle to penetrate calcified cartilage. Penetration through pyriform mucosa, carotid artery, or jugular vein is a theoretical risk in patients with unfavorable anatomy, although in practice it has not been reported.

Transthyrohyoid Vocal Fold Injection

The transthyrohyoid membrane VFI is a percutaneous approach that also uses an extramucosal route to the vocal fold.

- With this approach, a needle inserted through the thyrohyoid membrane is visualized intraluminally via flexible laryngoscopy and directed to the true vocal folds for injection. Anesthesia is similar to that for the other percutaneous approaches. However, after injection of the subcutaneous tissues, the needle is inserted through the thyrohyoid membrane, directed sharply caudal, and advanced until it is visualized penetrating the petiole of the epiglottis. Topical lidocaine can be injected onto the adducted vocal folds via this needle insertion to achieve laryngeal anesthetic.

- This needle is then withdrawn and replaced with a 25-gauge or 23-gauge needle attached to a syringe with the injection material.
- Again, once through the skin overlying the thyroid notch, the needle is directed caudally at a level nearly perpendicular to horizontal, and advanced until it is visualized intraluminally above the level of the anterior commissure.
- The needle is directed posteriorly and inserted in the posterior membranous vocal fold, just laterally to the thyroarytenoid muscle (**Fig. 3**C).
- Bending the needle, while improving the inferior angle, often makes directing the needle more difficult, and therefore is discouraged.[15]

Advantages and disadvantages of transthyrohyoid approach

The transthyrohyoid technique is unique in combining a percutaneous approach with direct visualization of needle placement within the lumen. As with other percutaneous approaches, the trajectory is easily reproducible in patients with favorable anatomy. Similarly, it is useful in patients who cannot tolerate peroral injection. When compared with other percutaneous techniques, precision is better with direct visualization of the needle tip, although obtaining optimal control is technically more challenging.

Transnasal, Endoscopic Vocal Fold Injection

The transnasal, endoscopic VFI uses a 23-gauge or 25-gauge flexible needle introduced through the working channel of the flexible laryngoscope.

- Anesthesia and patient positioning proceeds in identical fashion to the peroral approach.
- Injection material is primed through the tubing of the flexible needle, and the needle is then introduced through the working channel until it is visible beyond the tip of laryngoscope.
- The surgeon can vary the length of the needle extending beyond the laryngoscope, and then use the laryngoscope to direct the needle to the appropriate position under direct visualization. Injection results can similarly be assessed, as with other techniques.
- To date, the approach has been described for use with dilute collagen, either Cymetra with 2.3 mL of 1% lidocaine or Zyplast with 0.3% lidocaine.
- Because of the "memory" involved in the injection apparatus, small amounts of material will continue to flow after releasing pressure on the injection syringe.
- In addition, constant forward pressure must be maintained on the needle and laryngoscope while injecting, to overcome backpressure and displacement of the needle tip.
- Finally, because diluted collagen is used, 20% to 40% volume reduction with solvent absorption can be expected.[16,17]

Advantages and disadvantages of transnasal endoscopic approach

Advocates describe this technique as an alternative to other approaches for its ease of use, patient tolerance, and ability to overcome anatomic limitations. However, it should be noted that the fine-gauge injection needles only accommodate dilute preparations of most substances unless a high-pressure injection device is used. Also, because of the length of the flexible injection needle, this approach requires more than the normal amount of injection material to accommodate the relatively large dead space in the tubing. An additional drawback is that freedom of motion of the injection needle is limited, and essentially coupled to the laryngoscope; visualization centered away from the point of injection, which is beneficial in viewing augmentation of the medial edge, is not possible.

Superficial Vocal Fold Injection

Superficial VFI may be performed through the peroral, transthyrohyoid, or transnasal endoscopic approaches.

- The initial preparation and anesthetic are identical to the approaches used for deep VFI.
- Typically, methylprednisone 40 mg/mL for a total volume of 0.1 to 0.2 mL is used to treat subacute vocal fold scar.
- Collagen preparations may be used similarly to address focal lamina propria deficits or vocal fold scar.
- In all of the approaches, the needle is directed toward the area of interest and inserted submucosally.
- Test injection will reveal elevation of the epithelium, indicating infiltration of the Reinke space.
- The injection can then proceed until the target area has been infiltrated sufficiently.
- Because vocal fold scar is often tethered to the deeper layers of the lamina propria or vocal ligament, infiltration under a segment of tethered scar may not be possible with injection alone. For focal superficial injection, the precision afforded by peroral technique makes this an ideal approach.

IMMEDIATE POSTPROCEDURAL CARE

Immediate postprocedural care for office-based VFI requires a short period of observation. In uncomplicated cases, patients are observed for 15 to 30 minutes for signs or symptoms of respiratory distress, airway compromise, skin hematoma, or epistaxis. Because laryngeal anesthetic may increase propensity for aspiration, patients are instructed not to eat or drink for 1 to 2 hours after the procedure. Some advocate absolute or relative voice rest for the first 24 hours following the VFI. However, this is not universally practiced, and the potential benefits of avoiding superficial hemorrhage and premature material extrusion have not been substantiated by systematic studies.

POTENTIAL COMPLICATIONS AND MANAGEMENT

Among the most commonly encountered complications are failure to complete the procedure owing to inability to visualize vocal folds, excessive secretions, and/or gag reflex. More rarely, and often unreported, are complications of paraglottic hematoma, subepithelial hemorrhage, aspiration pneumonia, and airway compromise.

Failure to complete the procedure is the most commonly encountered complication with office-based VFI, and is reported at rates of 5% or less. This failure results most frequently from copious secretions, pain, or a strong gag reflex that cannot be overcome.

Also reported is the inability to properly visualize the vocal folds secondary to anatomy (usually overhanging arytenoid) or endoscope-related issues (inability to obtain proper angle of visualization). Visualization difficulties often cannot be overcome. In patients who cannot tolerate one approach, typically peroral, other approaches may be used, with good success rates.[11]

Excessive secretions may be prevented by avoiding excess topical anesthetic, and managed by oral suctioning and waiting for anesthetic to partially decrease the effect. A strong gag reflex can be managed by administering an additional 4% lidocaine or benzocaine perorally, although in some patients this may not be effective.

Less frequently reported reasons for aborted procedures include vasovagal syncope, vocal fold hematoma caused by the injection needle, and laryngeal edema on initial inspection.

The remaining complications from office-based VFIs are minor and infrequently reported.

Paraglottic hematoma has been reported with the trans-thyroid cartilage approach, and has been successfully observed.[12]

Subepithelial hemorrhage may also be observed, although some advocate treating with oral corticosteroids and strict voice rest when this occurs in professional voice users.

Aspiration pneumonia secondary to laryngeal anesthesia is a potential risk but has not been reported.

Airway compromise from overinjection, hemorrhage, or edema is a theoretical risk, and is rarely reported. Despite this, suspicion should remain high with a low threshold for reassessment and observation. Repeat endoscopy to ensure patent airway, inpatient admission if warranted, intravenous or oral corticosteroids, humidified oxygen, helium-oxygen mixtures, and nebulized racemic epinephrine are all mainstays for potential airway compromise.

Voice Worsening

Unintended superficial injection during deep VFI can have untoward effects on voice outcomes. To date, no commercially available material exists that replicates the rheological properties of the native superficial lamina propria. In addition, all injection materials induce inflammation to some degree. When these factors are combined, VFI into the superficial lamina propria can lead to severe impairment of vocal fold vibration acutely, and theoretically can induce scar formation in the chronic setting. This aspect is less concerning with the collagen-based products, which can be used as lamina propria replacements in scarred vocal folds. Superficial injection with other temporary substances, such as carboxymethylcellulose and hyaluronic acid, may also not be deleterious in the long term; the former anecdotally has been observed with no long-term effects, and the latter has been removed at 5 months postinjection with a return to baseline voice.[18] Concern for long-term effects of superficial injection are highest with calcium hydroxylapatite, as this material may produce greater inflammation, is significantly less pliable, and has a longer duration of integration than the temporary substances. Superficial injection with calcium hydroxylapatite is reported at rates of less than 1%. Worsening of voice, evidence for superficial injection, and markedly impaired mucosal wave are hallmark features of this complication. This anomaly may be corrected with lateral cordotomy, microflap elevation, and removal of the material, with good voice results.[19]

REHABILITATION AND RECOVERY

The immediate and long-term postoperative course following office-based VFI is typically uncomplicated and requires no definite adjuvant treatment. Immediate voice rest following VFI is controversial, although some advocate relative or absolute voice rest following deep VFI for 24 hours. Postprocedural antibiotics or corticosteroids are not routinely warranted. In uncomplicated cases, anticoagulation may be continued after the procedure. Postinjection patients may experience an acute worsening of voice with voice strain that lasts up to 5 days; this may be due to intended overinjection, minor hemorrhage and inflammation, and preexisting maladaptive laryngeal mechanics. If benefit is to be obtained, it may be delayed up to 5 to 7 days after injection, although this is not absolute. In addition, there is sparse literature regarding postinjection speaking-voice therapy; it is reasonable to surmise that postinjection voice therapy may benefit patients with long-standing conditions, such as vocal fold atrophy, or patients with preexisting laryngeal hyperfunction.

Postinjection swallowing results have been more disappointing, and may be more likely to require swallow therapy. In patients with unilateral vocal fold immobility, aspiration continues after VFI in 30% to 50% of patients, and is associated with decreased laryngeal elevation, delayed pharyngeal transit, and pharyngeal bolus residue.[20,21] Aspiration is higher in patients with multiple cranial neuropathies, concurrent neurologic disease, and high vagal injury.[22,23] Postinjection aspiration is as likely to occur after swallow as during a swallow, pointing to a multifactorial cause for dysphagia that goes beyond simple glottal incompetence.[20] Dysphagia in this patient population is closely related to pharyngeal strength, laryngeal elevation, and laryngeal sensitivity; as such, swallow evaluation with videofluoroscopy or flexible endoscopic evaluation of swallowing should be performed routinely. When warranted, swallow therapy should be instituted.

OUTCOMES WITH OFFICE-BASED VFI

There are several voice outcomes that are pertinent after office-based VFI. Subjectively, patients may note an improvement in volume, dyspnea with speaking, phonation time, voice strain, and vocal fatigue. Quantified outcomes may be reported in the form of patient-based questionnaires such as the voice handicap index (VHI), voice handicap index-10 (VHI-10), and voice-related quality-of-life score (V-RQOL). Subjective assessments made by independent observers, typically speech language pathologists, may include the Grade, Roughness, Breathiness, Asthenia, Strain (GRBAS) and Consensus Auditory Perceptual Evaluation—Voice (CAPE-V). Vocal function tests may include mean phonation time, mean phonation airflow, and fundamental frequency. Videostroboscopy may indicate improvement in position and augmentation of the vocal folds, glottic closure pattern, and no change or improvement in the mucosal wave. Though relevant clinically, the sum total of these parameters has rarely been reported in the literature, and is summarized in the next section.

Swallowing outcomes similarly may include subjective or objective parameters. Subjectively, patients may note improvement with aspiration symptoms and improved ability to clear secretions. Objectively, videofluoroscopy and flexible endoscopic evaluation of swallowing remain the mainstays of diagnosis, with particular attention to the Penetration Aspiration Scale (PAS). Ultimately, reinstitution of complete oral nutrition is the goal, and this, along with feeding-tube dependence, are often reported as outcome measures.

CLINICAL RESULTS IN THE LITERATURE

Voice outcomes after office-based VFI are generally favorable and comparable with those after VFI performed under microsuspension or direct laryngoscopy.[10,12] Voice outcomes with different materials show comparable results, with most studies showing some form of improvement in greater than 75% of patients. Regardless of the approach or material chosen, improvements in subjective voice perception, patient-based quality-of-life scores, blinded perceptual analysis, and/or stroboscopic parameters have been reported after office-based deep VFI.[5,10–12,15–18,24–26] Comparison across studies is difficult, as individual reports use disparate techniques and outcome measures and include different proportions of office-based versus operative VFI. Few studies independently look at voice outcomes with specific indications, although patients with paralysis and paresis potentially show greater improvement.[26] Recent evidence does suggest that early injection for unilateral vocal fold paralysis decreases the need for permanent medialization.[27–29] To date there are no studies that compare office-based VFI with medialization laryngoplasty. The presented studies are the largest series to include at least 50% office-based injections (**Table 1**).

Table 1
Vocal fold injection studies

Material	Study	No. of Patients	Duration of Follow-Up (mo)	Duration of Efficacy (mo)	Voice Results	Complications
CMC (Radiesse Voice Gel)	Mallur et al,[26] 2012	60	2.7	2.7	75% with improvement in VHI-10	None
Collagen (Cymetra)	Tan et al,[31] 2010	381	6–15	<6–15	n/a	4
HA (Restylane)	Song et al,[18] 2010	27	n/a	n/a	87% with subjective improvement	1
	Lau et al,[30] 2010	8	6	1–3	59.5% decrease in VHI score at 1 mo	1
CaHA (Radiesse Voice)	Rosen et al,[4] 2009	63	12	12	81% with subjective improvement at 12 mo	1
	Carroll and Rosen,[25] 2011	20	24	18.6	ΔVHI-10 of 10.7	3
	Rees et al,[24] 2008	51	5	5	ΔVHI-10 of 13.11	2

Abbreviations: CaHA, calcium hydroxylapatite; CMC, carboxymethyl cellulose; HA, hyaluronic acid; n/a, no data available; VHI, voice handicap index; VHI-10, voice handicap index-10.

Swallowing outcomes after VFI have been less favorable. Results have been disparate, although persistent aspiration after injection for unilateral vocal fold paralysis may be seen in 20% to 40% of patients.[19–21] The incidence is likely higher in patients with multiple cranial neuropathies or skull base lesions. Of the studies reported, 2 included patients who underwent office-based and operative VFI whereas 1 included patients who underwent office-based VFI only. Although frank aspiration is a concern, patients with hypomobility and atrophy may show poor pharyngeal transit, in part because of decreased swallowing pressures from glottal insufficiency. Future study looking at swallowing outcomes in this population is warranted.

SUMMARY

Office-based VFI has emerged as an efficacious, convenient, and cost-effective treatment for patients with glottal insufficiency. Techniques and materials vary, although reported outcomes are favorable regardless of approach or injection material. Complications are low and voice outcomes are comparable with those after injection performed under microsuspension laryngoscopy. Successful outcomes require familiarity with the specific approach and preprocedural planning. The potential for improvement, avoidance of general anesthesia, and low complication rates have made office-based VFI the standard of care for select patients with glottal insufficiency.

ACKNOWLEDGMENTS

The authors would like to thank Lucian Sulica, MD for providing artwork adapted for **Fig. 1**.

REFERENCES

1. Mau T, Brewer JM, Gatzert ST, et al. Three-dimensional conformation of the injected bolus in vocal fold injections in a cadaver model. Otolaryngol Head Neck Surg 2011;144(4):552–7.
2. Mau T, Weinheimer KT. Three-dimensional arytenoid movement induced by vocal fold injections. Laryngoscope 2010;120(8):1562–8.
3. Sulica L, Rosen CA, Postma GN, et al. Current practice in injection augmentation of the vocal folds: indications, treatment principles, techniques, and complications. Laryngoscope 2010;120(2):319–25.
4. Rosen CA, Amin MR, Sulica L, et al. Advances in office-based diagnosis and treatment in laryngology. Laryngoscope 2009;119:S185–214.
5. Carroll TL, Rosen CA. Trial vocal fold injection. J Voice 2010;24(4):494–8.
6. Burns JA, Friedman AD, Lutch MJ, et al. Subepithelial vocal fold infusion: a useful diagnostic and therapeutic technique. Ann Otol Rhinol Laryngol 2012;12(4): 224–30.
7. Martinex AA, Remacle M, Lawson G. Treatment of vocal fold scar by carbon dioxide laser and collagen injection: retrospective study on 12 patients. Eur Arch Otorhinolaryngol 2010;267(9):1409–14.
8. Mortensen M, Woo P. Office steroid injections of the larynx. Laryngoscope 2006; 116(10):1735–9.
9. Chhetri DK, Berke GS. Injection of cultured autologous fibroblasts for human vocal fold scars. Laryngoscope 2011;121(4):785–92.
10. Bove MJ, Jabbour N, Krishna P, et al. Operating room versus office-based injection laryngoplasty: a comparative analysis of reimbursement. Laryngoscope 2007;117(2):226–30.

11. Young VN, Smith LJ, Sulica L, et al. Patient tolerance of awake, in-office laryngeal procedures: a multi-institutional perspective. Laryngoscope 2012;122(2):315–21.
12. Mathison CC, Villari CR, Klein AM, et al. Comparison of outcomes and complications between awake and asleep injection laryngoplasty: a case-control study. Laryngoscope 2009;119(7):1417–23.
13. Tirado Y, Lewin JS, Hutcheson KA, et al. Office-based injection laryngoplasty in the irradiated larynx. Laryngoscope 2010;120(4):703–6.
14. Mallur PS, Rosen CA. Optimal visualization techniques for in-office and operative laryngologic procedures. Op Tech Otolaryngol, 2012;23(3):197–202.
15. Amin MR. Thyrohyoid approach for vocal fold augmentation. Ann Otol Rhinol Laryngol 2006;115(9):699–702.
16. Trask DK, Shellenberger DL, Hoffman HT. Transnasal, endoscopic vocal fold augmentation. Laryngoscope 2005;115(12):2262–5.
17. Pratap R, Mehta P, Blagnys B, et al. Early results for treatment of unilateral vocal fold palsy with injection medialisation under local anaesthetic. J Laryngol Otol 2009;123(8):873–6.
18. Song PC, Sung CK, Franco RA Jr. Voice outcomes after endoscopic injection laryngoplasty with hyaluronic acid stabilized gel. Laryngoscope 2010;120(Suppl 4): S199.
19. Chheda NN, Rosen CA, Belafsky PC, et al. Revision laryngeal surgery for the suboptimal injection of calcium hydroxylapatite. Laryngoscope 2008;118(12):2260–3.
20. Nayak VK, Bhattacharyya N, Kotz T, et al. Patterns of swallowing failure following medialization in unilateral vocal fold immobility. Laryngoscope 2002;112(10): 1840–4.
21. Bhattacharyya N, Kotz T, Shapiro J. Dysphagia and aspiration with unilateral vocal cord immobility: incidence, characterization, and response to surgical treatment. Ann Otol Rhinol Laryngol 2002;111(8):672–9.
22. Damrose EJ. Percutaneous injection laryngoplasty in the management of acute vocal fold paralysis. Laryngoscope 2010;120(8):1582–90.
23. Fang TJ, Tam YY, Courey MS, et al. Unilateral high vagal paralysis: relationship of the severity of swallowing disturbance and types of injuries. Laryngoscope 2011; 121(2):245–9.
24. Rees CJ, Mouadeb DA, Belafsky PC. Thyrohyoid vocal fold augmentation with calcium hydroxylapatite. Otolaryngol Head Neck Surg 2008;128(6):743–6.
25. Carroll TL, Rosen CA. Long-term results of calcium hydroxylapatite for vocal fold augmentation. Laryngoscope 2011;121(2):313–9.
26. Mallur PS, Morrison MP, Postma GN, et al. Safety and efficacy of carboxymethylcellulose in the treatment of glottic insufficiency. Laryngoscope 2012;122(2): 322–6.
27. Yung KC, Likhterov I, Courey MS. Effect of temporary vocal fold injection medialization on the rate of permanent medialization laryngoplasty in unilateral vocal fold paralysis patients. Laryngoscope 2011;121(10):2191–4.
28. Friedman AD, Burns JA, Heaton JT, et al. Early versus late injection medialization for unilateral vocal cord paralysis. Laryngoscope 2010;120(10):2042–6.
29. Young VN, Smith LJ, Rosen CA. Voice outcomes following acute unilateral vocal fold paralysis. Ann Otol Rhinol Laryngol 2012 [in press].
30. Lau DP, Lee GA, Wong SM, et al. Injection laryngoplasty with hyaluronic acid for unilateral vocal cord paralysis. Randomized controlled trial comparing two different particle sizes. J Voice 2010;24(1):113–8.
31. Injection laryngoplasty with micronized dermis: a 10-year experience with 381 injections in 344 patients. Laryngoscope 2010;120(12):2460–6.

Index

Note: Page numbers of article titles are in **boldface** type.

A

Airway dilation procedures, airway rupture and, 71
    deep tracheal lacerations and, 71
Airway surgery, ambulatory, outcomes of, 71–73
    dilatational methods in, 8
    office-based, **63–74**
        clinical results in literature, 72
        complications and management of, 69–71
        indications for, 64
        preoperative planning for, 64–65
        preparation and patient positioning for, 65–66
        procedural approach for, 66–69
        rehabilitation and recovery following, 71
Allyn, Welch, 6
Anesthesia, for office procedures, **13–19**
        approaches for, 13–14
        background of, 13
        patient selection for, 14–15
        postprocedure care and, 18
        safety and monitoring of, 18
        transnasal approach for, 14
        transoral approach for, 14
    topical, for office procedures, safety of, 15–18
Arnold, G.E., 6–7

B

Babington, Benjamin, 2
Balloon tracheoplasty, 66–69
Barrett's esophagus, transnasal esophagoscopy in, 43
Benedict, Edward, 5
Botulinum toxin, action of, 53
    serotypes of, 53–54
Botulinum toxin injections, contraindications to, 55
    inappropriate injection of, muscle weakness in, 59
    indications for, 54
    office-based, **53–61**
        complications of, 59
    outcomes and clinical results in literature, 59–60
    preoperative planning, preparation, and patient positioning for, 55
    procedural approach to, 55–59
    rehabilitation and recovery following, 59

Otolaryngol Clin N Am 46 (2013) 101–106
http://dx.doi.org/10.1016/S0030-6665(12)00194-6
oto.theclinics.com
0030-6665/13/$ – see front matter

Botulinum (*continued*)
  systemic effects of, 59
Bozzini, Philip, 2
Bronchoscopy, 66
Broyles, Edwin, 4

C

Cancer, of head and neck, transnasal esophagoscopy in, clinical results of, from literature, 43–44
Casserius, Julio, 2
Charge-coupled device, 6
Cinematography, high-speed, in voice disorders, 27–28
Cricopharyngeus muscle, injection of, 58–59
Czermak, Johann, 3

D

Dedo, H.H., 5, 7
Desormeaux, Antonin, 3
Dumon, J.F., 7
Dysphagia, morbidity and mortality associated with, 31–32

E

Edison, Thomas, 3
Endoscope, flexible, in evaluation of swallowing. See *Swallowing, flexible endoscopic evaluation of.*
  rigid, in laryngoscopy, 25
Endoscopy, contemporary office-based, beginning of, 5–6
  conventional, and transnasal esophagoscopy, compared, 42
  direct, advent of, 3–4
  early years of, 2–3
  flexible, 6–8
  in optical era, 4
  nasal, 15
Esophagoscopy, transnasal, **41–52**
    anatomic considerations for, 45–46
    and conventional endoscopy, compared, 42
    clinical results of, from literature, 48–49
    contraindications to, 44
    diagnostic applications of, 41
    immediate postprocedure care in, 46
    in Barrett's esophagus, 43
    in head and neck cancer, 43–44
    in *Helicobacter pylori*, 43
    in management of foreign bodies, 43
    in nasopharyngeal stenosis and neoplaryngeal stricture, 43
    indications for, 42–44
    level of examination using, 41
    outcomes of, 50

patient preparation and positioning for, 44
potential complications of, 47
preoperative planning for, 44
procedural approach for, 44–45

F

Flexible endoscope. See *Endoscope, flexible*.
Flexible endoscopy, 6–8
Flexible fiberoptic gastroscope, 6
Flexible fiberoptic laryngoscope, 6
Flexible laryngoscope, in laryngoscopy, 24–25
Foreign bodies, management of, transnasal esophagoscopy in, 43
Franco, R.A., 7

G

Garcia, Manuel, 2
Glottal leukoplakia/dysplasia, laser treatment of, 80
Green, Horace, 3
Gruntzig balloon catheter, 8

H

Head and neck, cancer of, transnasal esophagoscopy in, clinical results of, from literature, 43–44
Helicobacter pylori, transnasal esophagoscopy in, 43
Hertz, A.E., 8
Hoarseness, diagnosis of, 29
Hoffman, Friedrich, 2
Hollinger flexible forceps, 6
Hopkins, Harold, 5

I

Indirect laryngoscopy, 24–26

J

Jackson, Chevalier, 4, 8
Jako, G.J., 4, 5

K

Killian, Gustav, 3–4
Kirstein, Alfred, 3
Koufman, J.A., 6
Kymography, in voice disorders, 28

L

Lamm, Heinrich, 5–6
Laryngeal diseases, office-based laser procedures in. See *Laser procedures, laryngeal, office-based*.
Laryngeal injections, office-based, **85–100**
Laryngeal procedures, office-based, complications of, 82
outcomes and clinical results in literature, 82
postprocedural care in, 81
procedural approach for, 81–82
Laryngeal surgery, office-based, laser technology in, 7–8
Laryngology, development of field of, 1–2
Laryngopharyngeal biopsy, panendoscopy, and tumor staging, 80–82
Laryngoscope, flexible, in laryngoscopy, 24–25
Laryngoscopy, and stroboscopy, and other tools for evaluation of voice disorders, **21–30**
depth perception in, 25
flexible laryngoscope in, 24–25
indirect, 24–26
larynx visualization in, 24
laser, 69
rigid endoscope in, 25
stroboscopy and, 25–26, 27
Larynx, visualization of, in laryngoscopy, 24
Laser laryngoscopy, 69
Laser procedures, laryngeal, office-based, **75–84**
complications of, 78–79
in laryngeal diseases, 75
outcomes and clinical results in literature, 79–80
postprocedure care in, 78
preoperative planning for, 76
preparation and patient positioning for, 76
procedural approach for, 76
rehabilitation and recovery following, 79
selection of laser for, 76–78
surgical technique for, 78
Laser technology, in office-based laryngeal surgery, 7–8
Laser treatment, in glottal leukoplakia/dysplasia, 80
in vascular ectasias, 80
Lidocaine, allergy to, 17
and tetracaine, 17–18
for office procedures, 16–17
methemoglobinemia from, 17
topical application of, 16
toxicity of, 16–17
Lynch, R.C., 4

M

MacKenzie, Morell, 3
Methemoglobinemia, from lidocaine, 17

N

Narrow band imaging, in voice disorders, 28–29
Nasal endoscopy, 15
Nasopharyngeal stenosis, transnasal esophagoscopy in, 43
Nasopharyngolaryngoscopy, 6
Neopharyngeal stricture, transnasal esophagoscopy in, 43

P

Papilloma, laser treatment of, 79, 80
PCA muscle, injection of, 56–57
Pharyngeal squeeze maneuver, as predictor of swallowing safety, 34
  food textures and, 35
  in evaluation of swallowing, 34–35
    pharyngeal strength and, 34
    reliability of, 34–35
  related to Zenker's diverticulum, 35
Plummer, Henry, 8
Procedures and techniques, development of, for office, **1–11**

R

Rees, C.J., 8
Rigid endoscope, in laryngoscopy, 25

S

Solis-Cohen, Jacob, 3
Storz, Karl, 5
Storz-Hoptins telescope, 5
Stroboscopy, and laryngoscopy, 25–26, 27
    and other tools for evaluation of voice disorders, **21–30**
Strong, Stuart, 7
Swallowing, flexible endoscopic evaluation of, 32–34
    aging effects on penetration/aspiration and, 33
    patient preparation and positioning for, 32–33
    technique of, 33–34
    with sensory testing, 35–37
      in acute neurologic patients, 37
      in bedridden or incapacitated patients, 36–37
  in-office evaluation of, **31–39**
  pharyngeal squeeze maneuver in evaluation of, 34–35

T

TA-LCA muscle complex, 55–56
Tan, O.T., 7
Tetracaine, and lidocaine, 17–18
  for office procedures, 17–18
  toxicity of, 17
Tracheobronchial dilation, superficial tears and, 70–71

Tracheoplasty, 69
balloon, 66–69
Tracheoscopy, 66
Transnasal esophagoscopy, 6
Tyndall, John, 5

V

Vascular ectasias, laser treatment in, 80
Vocal cord paralysis, botulinum toxin injections in, 54
Vocal fold injections, office-based, as variable alternative to microsuspension or deep laryngoscopy, 86–87
assessment of mental faculties of patient and, 87–88
assessment of physical and anatomic aspects of patient and, 87–88
clinical results in literature, 97–99
complications and management of, 95–96
deep, 85–86
immediate postpocedural care following, 95
outcomes with, 97
preoperative planning for, 87–88
preparation and patient positioning for, 88–89
procedural approach for, 90–95
rehabilitation and recovery following, 96–97
superficial, 86
voice outcomes following, 96
tolerance of, 88
percutaneous (transcricothyroid and transthyroid cartilage), 92–93
peroral, 90–92
studies of, 98
transnasal, endoscopic, 94
transthyrohyoid, 93–94
Vocal fold motion, paradoxic, 54
Vocal fold(s), false, 57–58
granulomas of, 54
Voice disorders, evaluation of, 22–24
high-speed cinematography in, 27–28
history taking in, 22–23
investigational techniques in, 27–29
kymography in, 28
laryngoscopy, stroboscopy, and other tools for evaluation of, **21–30**
narrow band imaging in, 28–29
voice examination in, 23–24
Voice production, diseases impacting on, 54

W

Ward, Paul, 7
Wolf-Schindler gastroscope, 5

Z

Zeiss Optical Company, 4
Zenker's diverticulum, pharyngeal squeeze maneuver and, 35

Moving?

Make sure your subscription
moves with you!

To notify us of your new address, find your Clinics Account
Number (located on your mailing label above your name),
and contact customer service at:

Email: journalscustomerservice-usa@elsevier.com

800-654-2452 (subscribers in the U.S. & Canada)
314-447-8871 (subscribers outside of the U.S. & Canada)

Fax number: 314-447-8029

Elsevier Health Sciences Division
Subscription Customer Service
3251 Riverport Lane
Maryland Heights, MO 63043

*To ensure uninterrupted delivery of your subscription,
please notify us at least 4 weeks in advance of move.*

Printed and bound by CPI Group (UK) Ltd, Croydon, CR0 4YY

03/10/2024

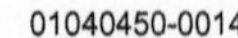

01040450-0014